£39.50

Radiological Atlas of Gastrointestinal Disease

Radiological Atlas of
Gastrointestinal
Disease

DANIEL J. NOLAN
MD MRCP FRCR
Consultant Radiologist, John Radcliffe Hospital, Oxford;
Clinical Lecturer, University of Oxford

with contributions by

STUART FIELD MA FRCR. *Consultant Radiologist, Department
of Diagnostic Radiology, Kent & Canterbury Hospital, Canterbury:*
DAVID J. ALLISON BSc MD FRCR. *Professor of Diagnostic
Radiology, Royal Postgraduate Medical School, Hammersmith
Hospital, London:*
ANNE P. HEMINGWAY BSc MRCP FRCR. *Senior Lecturer,
Department of Diagnostic Radiology, Royal Postgraduate Medical
School, Hammersmith Hospital, London*

Foreword by
EMANOEL C. G. LEE MCh FRCS(Edin) FRCS(Eng).
Consultant Surgeon, John Radcliffe Hospital, Oxford

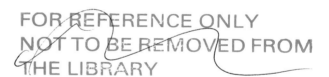
A Wiley Medical Publication

JOHN WILEY & SONS
Chichester · New York · Brisbane · Toronto · Singapore

Library of Congress Cataloging in Publication Data:

Nolan, Daniel J.
   Radiological atlas of gastrointestinal disease.
   (A Wiley medical publication)
   Includes index.
   1. Gastrointestinal system—Radiography.
   2. Gastrointestinal system—Diseases—Diagnosis. I. Field, Stuart. II. Allison, David J. III. Hemingway, Anne P. IV. Title. V. Series. [DNLM: 1. Gastrointestinal system—Radiography—Atlases. WI 17 N787r]
RC804.R6N65 1983   616.3'30757   82–13629

ISBN 0 471 25917 9

British Library Cataloguing in Publication Data:

Nolan, Daniel J.
   Radiological atlas of gastrointestinal disease.
   —(A Wiley medical publication)
   1. Alimentary canal   2. Radiology, Medical
   I. Title
   616.3'30757   RC860

ISBN 0 471 25917 9

Filmset by Eta Services (Typesetters) Ltd., Beccles, Suffolk.

Contents

Foreword

It is fitting that a surgeon or physician rather than a radiologist be asked to write an introduction to this Radiological Atlas of Gastrointestinal Disease. During the last two decades the association of physician, surgeon, radiologist and pathologist in so-called multi-disciplinary groups has been the main spur to the rapid developments in clinical gastroenterology. Improvements in radiological diagnosis have been at the forefront of these developments. This is especially true of the double-contrast barium examinations of the stomach and colon, and of the small-bowel enema investigations, which have played such a major role in the management of Crohn's disease. Dr. Nolan has been an innovator and developer in all these fields, and the Atlas which he and his colleagues have produced maintains the high standard he always sets for himself. The chapter dealing with Plain Films of the Acute Abdomen will be of particular use to the young surgeons on duty at night during the admission of emergency cases. However, it is the wide range of the diseases which are covered by the Atlas, and the expertise and excellent illustrations of disease process at each site, which make this book so useful to all clinicians with an interest in the gastrointestinal tract.

EMANOEL C.G. LEE

1983

Preface

Significant changes have taken place in the radiological techniques used to examine the gastrointestinal tract. The improved methods give adequate definition and evaluation of all segments of the tract and thus contribute very positively to the diagnosis and assessment of gastrointestinal disease.

Double-contrast barium studies are used routinely in most centres to examine the upper gastrointestinal tract and colon and have the advantages that the mucosal surface of the tract is shown *en face* and the radiological appearances closely resemble those seen by the naked eye.

The barium infusion technique for examining the small intestine has become easier with the more flexible tubes now available for intubation. Barium infused directly distends the small intestine, giving optimum visualization of any lesion that may be present; there is excellent correlation between the radiological appearances and the findings at morbid anatomy.

It is necessary to perform barium studies in the majority of patients suspected of having a disorder of the gastrointestinal tract. However, in some cases plain abdominal radiographs give sufficient information for a diagnosis to be made, whilst in others it may be necessary to proceed to angiography.

Disorders of the gastrointestinal tract are displayed in this atlas with particular emphasis upon the appearances elicited by the newer radiological techniques. Each chapter carries a short introduction, the illustrations are accompanied by explanatory captions in some detail, and there is a considerable bibliography. This well-illustrated atlas of gastrointestinal disease and guide to current radiographic methods will assist all those whose concern is with the diagnosis and management of gastrointestinal disease.

DANIEL J. NOLAN

1983

Acknowledgements

This book would be incomplete without the contributions of Dr. David Allison, Dr. Stuart Field and Dr. Anne Hemingway, and the many kind colleagues who have provided me with radiographs, all of whom I have endeavoured to acknowledge in the text. I am grateful to them and to the publishers and editors of journals who have allowed me to reproduce their material.

The high-quality radiography was provided by the radiographers at the Radcliffe Infirmary and the John Radcliffe Hospital.

I am indebted to my secretary, Miss Susan Dyson, and my wife Rosarie who prepared the manuscript, and to Mr. Patrick West of John Wiley & Sons for his invaluable assistance.

Radiological techniques play a major role in the investigation and management of gastrointestinal tract disease. Plain radiography can sometimes provide useful information. In the majority of cases, however, it is necessary to do barium studies of the upper gastrointestinal tract, small intestine or colon to obtain the required diagnostic information. Angiography and radionuclide studies are helpful, particularly in the investigation of obscure gastrointestinal bleeding. In this chapter a brief outline of the methods available for examining the gastrointestinal tract is given. Readers who require details of the different techniques are referred to the reference list.

1 The Gastrointestinal Tract— Radiological Investigation

Plain radiographs

Plain radiographs of the chest and abdomen are important in patients who present with symptoms and signs of an 'acute abdomen' as they may show evidence of perforation or obstruction. A description of the technique used for obtaining good quality plain abdominal radiographs is given in Chapter 2.

Barium studies

Upper gastrointestinal tract Barium studies of the upper gastrointestinal tract are indicated for patients who present with dysphagia, dyspepsia, anaemia, gastrointestinal bleeding, unexplained weight loss or a palpable mass in the upper abdomen.

The double-contrast barium technique is the method of choice for examining the oesophagus, stomach and duodenum, as lesions are shown *en face* and their size, shape and margins are clearly shown. Compression radiography and the filling method are included in the examination. The technique for performing double-contrast barium examinations has previously been described in detail (Shirakabe 1971; Kreel *et al.* 1973; Nolan 1980). The aim of the examination is to coat the mucosal surface of the stomach with an even coating of barium. Gas, in the form of effervescent tablets or granules, is taken to distend the stomach. Sufficient gas is used to put the gastric mucosa under slight tension so that lesions that lack distensibility such as ulcers, ulcer scars and carcinomas produce a clearly visible series of converging folds (Gelfand 1975). Smooth-muscle relaxants, hyoscine butylbromide (Buscopan) or glucagon, are administered so that the stomach and duodenum can be examined in a state of hypotonia.

The first film, a prone mucosal view of the anterior wall of the stomach, is obtained after the patient has swallowed a small amount of barium. More barium is taken and when adequate gas has been produced by the effervescent agent further radiographs are taken. The supine, supine right anterior oblique and supine left anterior oblique positions show the mucosal pattern of the antrum, body and fundus of the stomach. Double-contrast views of the duodenum are taken in the supine right anterior oblique and prone positions. A further mucosal view of the fundus is obtained with the head

1

of the table elevated to an angle of 45°. With the patient standing, compression is applied to the barium-filled stomach and duodenum and radiographs are taken if any abnormal feature is recognized. Good double-contrast views of the whole oesophagus can be obtained by getting the patient to drink the barium suspension while standing holding his nose. In this way large amounts of air are swallowed with the barium. Special attention is paid to examination of the oesophagus in patients with oesophageal symptoms. Views of the whole oesophagus, supplemented if necessary by rapid serial or cine radiography, are obtained. Constricting lesions of the oesophagus, stomach or duodenum are demonstrated better with the single-contrast column of barium than on double-contrast views. Patients who present with vomiting due to a suspected obstructing lesion are examined by the single-contrast barium method. A modified double-contrast examination is performed in patients who have had previous gastric surgery.

The duodenum as far as the ligament of Treitz is included in the routine double-contrast examination of the upper gastrointestinal tract. Hypotonic duodenography, as a separate study, is performed if the prime area of interest is the duodenal loop or the head of the pancreas. The intubation method gives consistently better results than the tubeless method, particularly in the investigation of suspected pancreatic lesions. Patients with obstructive jaundice are best examined by fine-needle percutaneous cholangiography and hypotonic duodenography performed as a combined procedure (Gourtsoyiannis & Nolan 1979).

Fibre-optic endoscopy is now widely used and makes it possible to visualize, photograph and obtain aimed biopsy and cytology specimens. It has been claimed that endoscopy is more accurate at detecting lesions in the gastrointestinal tract than the barium meal. This argument does not hold when proper double-contrast examinations are performed. The accuracy of both techniques depends on the expertise of the person performing the examination. The double-contrast method has a number of advantages: it is quick to perform, it is safer and more comfortable for the patient than endoscopy, and sedation is not required. Each radiograph provides an image of a large area of oesophagus, stomach or duodenum which is retained as a permanent record and is available at any time for detailed review.

Small intestine The follow-through is the most widely used procedure for examining the small intestine with barium and is normally performed following a barium meal examination of the oesophagus, stomach and duodenum. It is not accurate at detecting and demonstrating diseases that cause morphological changes of the small intestine. Duodenal intubation methods are more accurate and are replacing the follow-through in many centres (Nolan 1981). The single-contrast dilute barium infusion method described by Sellink (1971) is very satisfactory and in my opinion is the method of choice for routinely examining the small intestine with barium.

Barium examination is indicated for the investigation of known or suspected diseases of the small intestine such as Crohn's disease, tuberculosis, tumours, radiation damage and ischaemia. Unexplained abdominal pain, diarrhoea, weight loss and malabsorption are the most common presenting features of these conditions although they may also present as an 'acute abdomen' or unexplained anaemia. The infusion examination is also useful in the investigation of small intestinal obstruction (Nolan & Marks 1981). A jejunal biopsy is the initial investigation in patients with suspected coeliac disease and the barium infusion is used only if there is a suspected complication of coeliac disease such as lymphoma.

There are a number of other ways of examining the small intestine with barium. Patients with small intestinal obstruction may have barium injected through intestinal tubes, such as the Miller–Abbott or Cantor tube, which will outline the obstructing lesion. The terminal ileum can also be examined by refluxing barium through the ileocaecal valve during barium enema examination. Miller (1965) described a technique whereby the whole small intestine can be demonstrated by refluxing barium from the colon into the terminal ileum. This complete reflux technique is particularly useful in the investigation of small intestinal obstruction. Excellent visualization of the ileocaecal region can be obtained by administering barium orally, and when the head of the barium column reaches the terminal ileum air is introduced rectally—the per oral pneumocolon examination (Kellett et al. 1977).

The colon The double-contrast barium enema is the technique of choice for examining the colon as it is sensitive enough to detect small polyps of the colon as well as cancers (Nolan 1982). Most radiologists agree that the double-contrast method should be used routinely.

The main indications for performing a double-contrast barium enema are to detect colorectal cancer and polyps and in the diagnosis and management of inflammatory bowel disease. Bleeding per rectum, anaemia, change in bowel habit and weight loss are the most frequent presenting symptoms of these conditions. The barium examination is contraindicated if there is suspected perforation of the colon or toxic megacolon. If obstruction or complications of diverticular disease such as fistula formation are suspected, a single-contrast barium enema should be performed. The single-contrast examination can also help confirm the presence of a carcinoma of the caecum or ascending colon in cases where there is poor mucosal coating of the right side of the colon at double-contrast examination.

It is most important to obtain a clean colon before performing a barium enema examination. A combination of low residue diet, increased fluid intake, cathartics and a cleansing enema are essential for consistently getting the colon clean (Miller 1975). The barium suspension is introduced into the rectum under gravity and allowed to flow as far as the hepatic flexure. It is then drained off or the patient is sent to the toilet. A smooth-muscle relaxant such as 20 mg of hyoscine butylbromide (Buscopan) is injected intravenously and air is introduced per rectum so that as the head of the barium column advances to the caecum air distends the colon. The following views are then taken with the table horizontal: lateral of the rectum, right anterior oblique of the sigmoid colon, full-length prone, prone of the sigmoid colon with the tube angled caudad 30°, full-length supine, right decubitus and left decubitus. The patient is then brought upright and oblique views of the flexures are obtained. Spot views are taken as required.

The introduction and widespread use of fibre-optic colonoscopy has led to the more accurate assessment of polyps and colonic cancer. It is possible to remove polyps and to obtain biopsies from polypoid lesions and from the mucosa of the colon. However, lesions may be missed at the flexures because of sharp angulation and the colonoscopist fails to get the endoscope as far as the caecum in at least 10 per cent of cases. Digital examination, sigmoidoscopy and the barium enema remain the initial diagnostic procedures in patients with suspected colonic disease. Good double-contrast barium radiology and colonoscopy are complementary and their combined diagnostic accuracy exceeds that of either technique (Miller & Lehman 1978).

Water-soluble contrast studies

Plain abdominal radiography is the initial diagnostic procedure in patients with suspected perforation of the stomach or duodenum. If there is no evidence of free gas on the plain radiographs but perforation is still suspected, water-soluble contrast agents are used. The contrast medium should preferably be injected through a nasogastric tube directly into the stomach. Diatrizoate in the form of Gastrografin is more likely to produce local tissue reaction than other water-soluble contrast agents (Margulis 1977); it should only be used if it is being taken orally. Water-soluble contrast agents are hyperosmolar and will draw fluid into the lumen of the intestine. Their use can cause shock and possibly death, particularly in infants, children, the aged and the very ill (Margulis 1977). It is important, therefore, to monitor the fluid and electrolyte balance of patients at risk.

Water-soluble contrast studies are seldom helpful in the small intestine. They can be useful in the colon to establish if there is a leak or stenosis at the anastomosis site in patients who have had a sigmoid colectomy.

Angiography

Selective visceral angiography is invaluable in certain patients who present with bleeding from the gastrointestinal tract when more conventional techniques have failed to locate the bleeding site. Angiography is dealt with in more detail in Chapter 9.

Radionuclide studies

Radionuclide imaging can be useful in helping to detect and localize obscure bleeding sites in the small intestine and colon. Alavi (1980) recommends the use of freshly prepared ^{99m}Tc sulphur colloid which is administered by intravenous injection. The general anatomical location of the bleeding can be detected and further investigations such as barium studies or angiography are then performed to define the site precisely. Bleeding rates of as little as 0.05–0.1 ml/min can be detected by this method (Alavi 1980).

Patients with suspected Meckel's diverticulum should have radionuclide imaging performed using ^{99m}Tc-pertechnetate as the initial diagnostic procedure (Conway 1980). Meckel's diverticulum is shown as an area of increased radionuclide activity in the lower abdomen.

References

Alavi A. (1980) Scintigraphic demonstration of acute gastrointestinal bleeding. *Gastrointest. Radiol.*, **5**, 205

Conway J.J. (1980) Radionuclide diagnosis of Meckel's diverticulum. *Gastrointest. Radiol.*, **5**, 209

Gelfand D.W. (1975) The double contrast upper gastrointestinal examination in the Japanese style. *Am. J. Gastroenterol.*, **63**, 216

Gourtsoyiannis N.C. & Nolan D.J. (1979) Combined fine needle percutaneous transhepatic cholangiography and hypotonic duodenography in obstructive jaundice. *Clin. Radiol.*, **30**, 507

Kellett M.J., Zboralske F.F. & Margulis A.R. (1977) Per oral pneumocolon examination of the ileocaecal region. *Gastrointest. Radiol.*, **1**, 361

Kreel L., Herlinger H. & Glanville J. (1973) Technique of the double contrast barium meal with examples of correlation with endoscopy. *Clin. Radiol.*, **24**, 307

Margulis A.R. (1977) Water-soluble radiographic contrast agents in the gastrointestinal tract. In *Radiographic Contrast Agents* (Eds. Miller R.E. & Skucas J.). Baltimore: University Park Press

Miller R.E. (1965) Complete reflux small bowel examination. *Radiology*, **84**, 457

Miller R.E. (1975) The cleansing enema. *Radiology*, **117**, 483

Miller R.E. & Lehman G. (1978) Polypoid colonic lesions undetected by endoscopy. *Radiology*, **129**, 295

Miller R.E. & Sellink J.L. (1979) Enteroclysis: the small bowel enema. How to succeed and how to fail. *Gastrointest. Radiol.*, **4**, 269

Nolan D.J. (1980) *The Double-Contrast Barium Meal— A Radiological Atlas*. Aylesbury: HM + M

Nolan D.J. (1981) The barium examination of the small intestine. Progress report. *Gut*, **22**, 682

Nolan D.J. (1982) Radiological assessment. In *Recent Results in Cancer Research*, Vol. 83, *Colorectal Cancer* (Ed. Duncan W.). Berlin: Springer-Verlag

Nolan D.J. & Marks C.G. (1981) The barium infusion in small intestinal obstruction. *Clin. Radiol.*, **32**, 651

Op den Orth J.O. & Ploem S. (1975) The stalactite phenomenon in double contrast studies of the stomach. *Radiology*, **117**, 523

Sellink J.L. (1971) *Examination of the Small Intestine by Means of Duodenal Intubation*. Leiden: Stenfert Kroese BV

Sellink J.L. & Miller R.E. (1982) *Radiology of the Small Bowel—Modern Enteroclysis Technique and Atlas.* The Hague: Martinus Nijhoff

Shirakabe H. (1971) *Double Contrast Studies of the Stomach.* Tokyo: Bunkodo Company

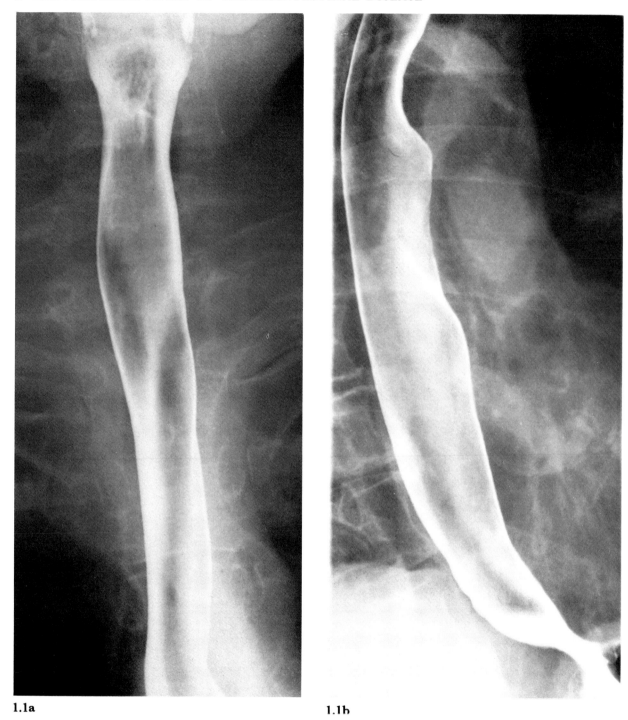

1.1a   **1.1b**

1.1 a,b *Double-contrast views* of the normal oesophagus

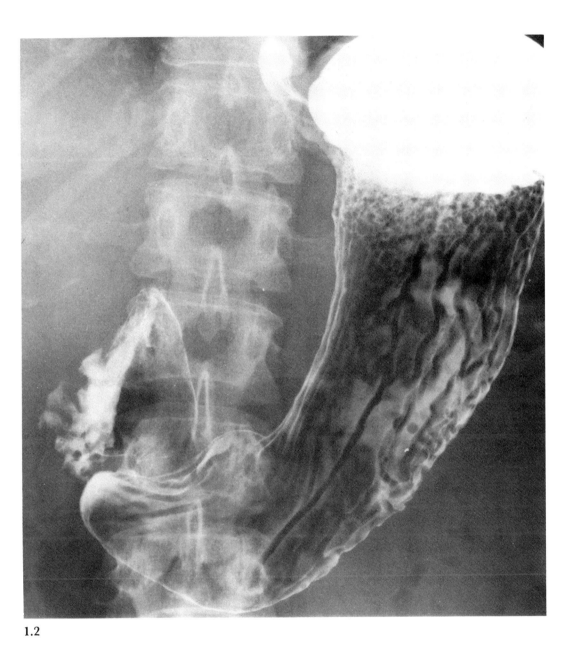

1.2

1.2 *Supine double-contrast view* showing the body and antrum of the stomach and the duodenal cap

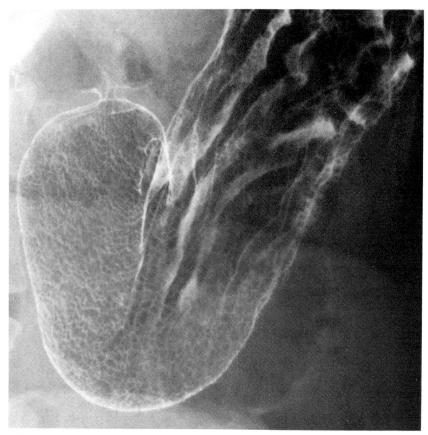

1.3

1.3 *Supine right anterior oblique double-contrast view* showing the antrum and body of the stomach. The fine mucosal detail—the areae gastricae—is clearly demonstrated

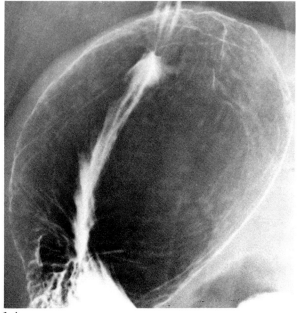

1.4

1.4 *Supine left anterior double-contrast view* showing the fundus of the stomach. The oesophagogastric junction is shown *en face* on this view with the patient in the lateral position

1.5 *Supine double-contrast view* showing the upper body of the stomach. The anterior wall mucosal folds show a 'tramline' appearance. A drop of barium is hanging from an anterior wall fold (arrow). This appearance has been called the stalactite phenomenon (Op den Orth & Ploem 1975) and should be distinguished from a small ulcer

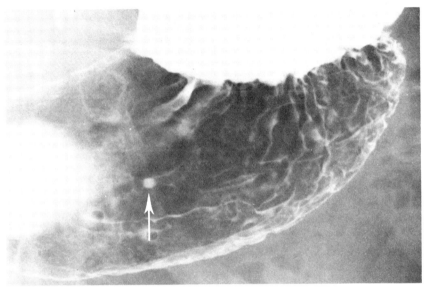

1.5

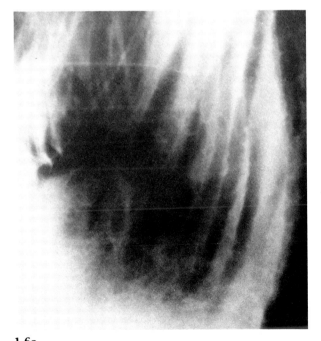

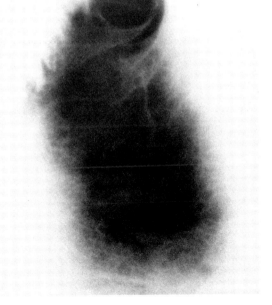

1.6a   **1.6b**

1.6 a,b *Spot compression views* of the barium-filled stomach showing the mucosal folds and the areae gastricae pattern

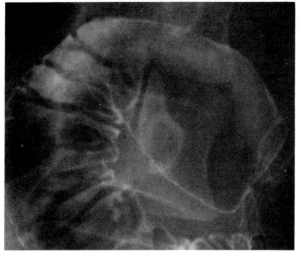

1.7

1.7 A *double-contrast view* of the duodenal cap

1.8 *Normal hypotonic double-contrast view* of the duodenal cap and loop

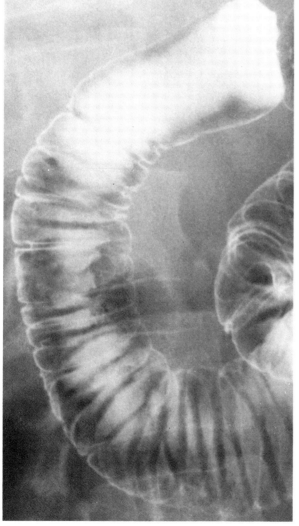

1.8

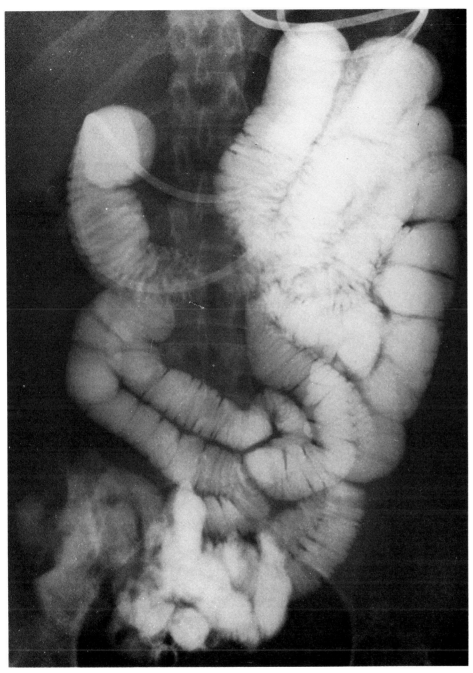

1.9

1.9 *Normal barium infusion examination* showing the small intestine outlined with barium

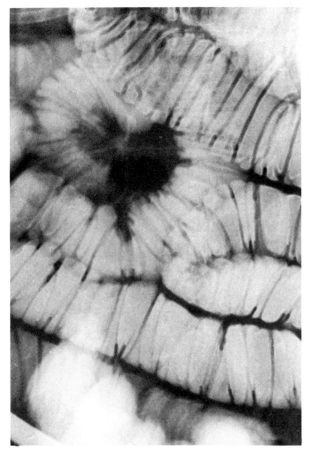

1.10a

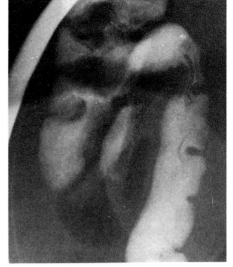

1.10b

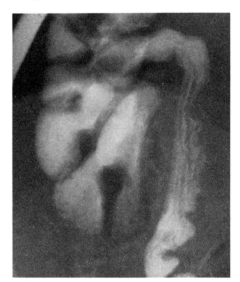

1.10c

1.10 **Normal ileum** a *Spot view* of loops of ileum. b,c *Spot views* of terminal ileum

1.11 *Peroral pneumocolon examination* showing the terminal ileum and caecum

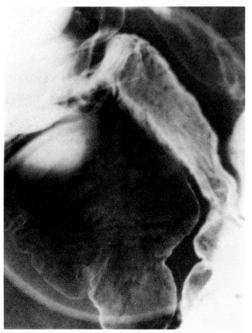

1.11

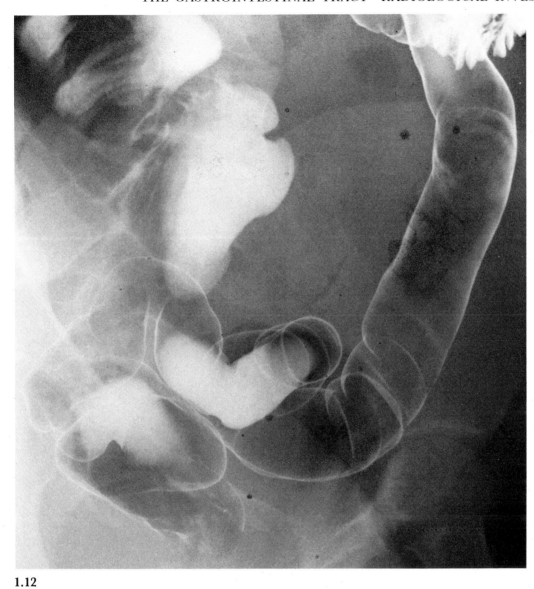

1.12

1.12 *Oblique double-contrast barium enema view* of the sigmoid colon and rectum

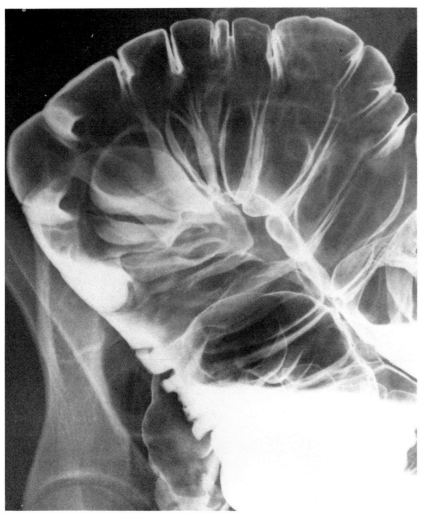

1.13a

1.13

1.13 a,b *Normal double-contrast views* of the hepatic and splenic flexures taken with the patient standing

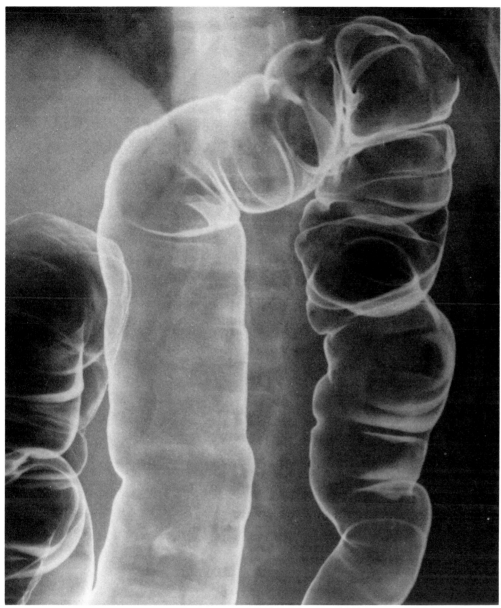

1.13b

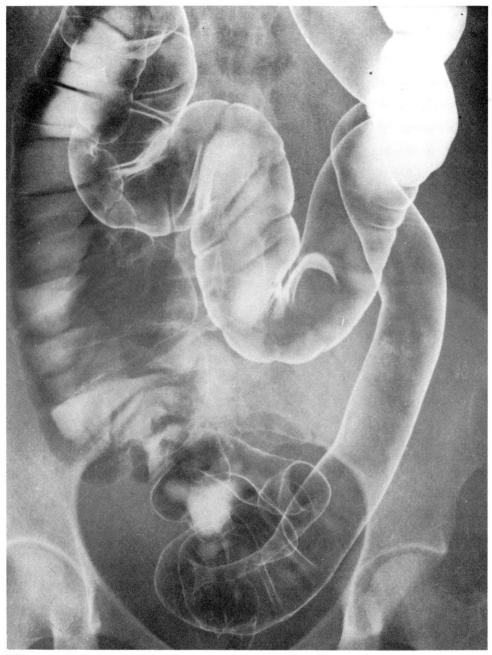

1.14

1.14 *Supine double-contrast view* of the colon and rectum

2 The Plain Film in the Acute Abdomen

Stuart Field

The interpretation of the plain abdominal X-ray in the clinical setting of an acute abdomen is a challenging task. Often a specific diagnosis can be made on the plain films and surgery indicated on this evidence alone. Sometimes further investigations using barium studies or ultrasound may be helpful. However, the radiological examination may be unhelpful and in these circumstances, if there are clinical indications for immediate surgery, negative or equivocal radiology should be ignored.

Radiographic technique

An erect PA chest and a supine abdomen can be regarded as the standard films. A horizontal beam abdominal film is usually taken to aid diagnosis further, but the significance of air/fluid levels in the bowel is frequently over-estimated. Gammill & Nice (1972) have stressed the normality of colonic air/fluid levels, some of which may be several centimetres in length, and, furthermore, air/fluid levels in the bowel do not help in distinguishing intestinal obstruction from paralytic ileus.

A chest radiograph is important because chest disease such as myocardial infarction, pulmonary infarction, dissecting aneurysm and pneumonia may simulate an 'acute' abdomen. It is also useful to have a chest radiograph as a baseline because post-operative chest complications and subphrenic abscess in patients with an acute abdomen are relatively frequent. An erect chest film is one of the best views to demonstrate free intra-abdominal gas and is superior to the erect abdomen. It takes time for free gas to accumulate and the patient should be sitting or standing for 10 minutes prior to the radiograph (Bryant et al. 1963). If this is not possible, then a right-side-up decubitus abdomen view, which will demonstrate gas between the liver and the lateral abdominal wall, is the film of choice.

Free intra-abdominal gas

Free intraperitoneal gas almost always indicates a perforated viscus, although only about 70 per cent of perforated peptic ulcers will demonstrate free gas and a perforated appendix almost never. As little as 1 ml of free gas can be demonstrated using a horizontal ray technique, either on an erect chest or a right-side-up lateral decubitus radiograph (Miller 1973). Radiographic technique is important, however, and it is stressed that a patient should remain in the position of the horizontal ray film for 5–10 minutes prior to the film being taken to allow any free gas present to rise to the highest position (Bryant et al. 1963).

A horizontal ray film—erect chest or decubitus abdomen— is mandatory for patients in whom a perforated viscus is suspected. There are many patients, particularly those critically ill, unconscious, following trauma, or elderly, in whom perforation of a viscus may be clinically silent as it is overshadowed by other serious medical or surgical problems. In

17

such patients a supine abdominal radiograph (frequently portable) is the only examination possible. It is very important, therefore, to recognize the signs of pneumoperitoneum in these films.

Free intra-abdominal gas can be detected on the supine abdominal radiograph in 56 per cent of patients (Menuck & Siemers 1976). The most common finding is a collection of intraperitoneal air in the right upper quadrant immediately adjacent to the liver and lying mainly in the right subhepatic space and Morrison's pouch (hepatorenal fossa). Other less common signs of free gas on supine radiographs are visualization of the outer wall of a loop of bowel, visualization of the falciform ligament, umbilical ligaments or the urachus.

It is important to recognize those patients in whom a pneumoperitoneum may occur without clinical evidence of perforation. The majority will have had a silent perforation but the others may have any one of a variety of conditions.

Pneumoperitoneum without peritonitis

perforated peptic ulcer or viscus, which has sealed itself, in old people, coma, patients on respirators, patients on steroids, patients with any other serious medical condition;
perforated jejunal diverticulosis;
perforated cyst in pneumatosis intestinalis;
stercoral ulceration;
tracking down from a pneumomediastinum;
leakage through a distended stomach (e.g. endoscopy);
vaginal-tubal entry of air;
post-operative;
peritoneal dialysis.

Post-operative gas

In the event of a post-operative complication it may be necessary to differentiate between residual air from the operation, gas from an abscess, or leak from a gastrointestinal tract anastomosis. Post-operative gas may be present for up to four weeks. Important factors influencing the rate of disappearance are the amount of air present initially and the body habitus—air remaining longer in thinner patients. However, no factor is reliable in predicting either the presence or duration of post-operative gas in a given patient.

The presence of free gas in obese patients beyond the fourth post-operative day is usually of major clinical significance. Increasing volumes of gas are also significant, providing the positioning and radiographic technique is identical, and the presence

of intra-abdominal drains has been considered (Bryant et al. 1963).

A number of conditions may simulate free intra-abdominal gas and it is very important to distinguish these from true pneumoperitoneum. Failure to do so may well result in an unnecessary laparotomy.

Conditions simulating pneumoperitoneum

intestine between liver and diaphragm;
linear pulmonary collapse;
subphrenic abscess;
subdiaphragmatic fat;
cysts in pneumatosis intestinalis;
small diaphragmatic hump.

Intestinal obstruction

The amount of gas and fluid normally present in the alimentary tract of any individual is very variable. Relatively large amounts of gas are usually present in the stomach and colon; fluid levels are commonly seen in the stomach, duodenum and colon. The presence of more than two fluid levels greater than 2.5 cm in length in the small bowel indicates abnormality, usually obstruction or paralytic ileus (Gammill & Nice 1972). Unfortunately there is no agreed upper limit of normal for the diameter of the large bowel although 5.5 cm has been suggested; above this megacolon should be diagnosed in inflammatory bowel disease (Hywel Jones & Chapman 1969). There is considerable overlap between normal and abnormal; it varies greatly with age and some patients with obstructed colons have smaller colon diameters than many normal people.

Dilatation of the bowel occurs in both mechanical obstruction and paralytic ileus. The radiological differentiation depends mainly on the distribution and relative size of the dilated loops (Table 2.1). With the exception of the presence of solid faeces, the distinguishing signs between small and large bowel dilatation are sometimes misleading. Problems in distinguishing lower ileum from sigmoid are relatively frequent—both may be smooth in outline and occupy a similar position low in the abdomen. Mechanical obstruction of the small bowel causes small bowel dilation with reduced calibre of the large bowel. The 'string of beads' sign is very useful because it is highly suggestive of small bowel obstruction (Figure 2.13). It is caused by air trapped between the bands of valvulae conniventes in the dilated, mainly fluid-filled, small bowel. Dilated bowel usually contains some gas but occasionally it is only fluid-filled and then it is very difficult to assess the bowel calibre.

Table 2.1 Distinction between large and small bowel dilatation

	Small bowel	Large bowel
Distribution	Central	Peripheral
Number of loops	Many	Few
Solid faeces	Absent	Present
Haustra	Absent	Present in ascending colon and transverse colon. May be absent in descending and sigmoid colon
Valvulae conniventes	Present in jejunum	Absent
Radius of curvature of loop	Small	Large

Distal large bowel obstruction and paralytic ileus may be indistinguishable on plain radiographs, both resulting in dilatation of small and large bowel. Proximal large bowel obstruction causes dilatation up to the point of obstruction although ischaemic colitis can cause similar appearances. The specific cause of intestinal obstruction can only infrequently be made from the radiograph but includes strangulated hernia and gallstone ileus. A specific diagnosis can often be made if obstruction is due to a closed loop such as gastric volvulus, small bowel volvulus, caecal volvulus or sigmoid volvulus.

Volvulus

Gastric volvulus is rare, but the presence of a grossly dilated stomach with no bowel gas beyond is fairly typical. Small bowel volvulus is not uncommon; however, the closed loop may be fluid-filled and difficult to identify. Even if the closed small bowel loop is gas-filled it is often difficult to distinguish it from the remaining dilated small bowel, and specific diagnosis is impossible. Occasionally small bowel volvulus is seen with the characteristic 'coffee bean' appearance.

Caecal or right colon volvulus can only occur when there is a degree of malrotation and the caecum and ascending colon are on a mesentery. The caecum, in about half such cases, becomes twisted and inverted so that the pole of the caecum and appendix occupy the left upper quadrant. In the other half, twist without inversion occurs and the caecum still occupies the right half of the abdomen, usually the right lower quadrant. In spite of considerable distension of the volved caecum it is usual for one or two haustral markings to remain. The distended caecum may be readily identified or partly obscured by marked gas/fluid distension of the small bowel.

Volvulus of the sigmoid colon is the most common type of volvulus and is almost always caused by twisting of the sigmoid loop around its mesenteric axis. Although a specific diagnosis can often be made on the plain radiograph, up to one-third of cases are diagnostically difficult (Young et al. 1978). The diagnosis depends on identifying the loop of sigmoid which usually has an ahaustral margin, an apex on the left above the level of D10 and an inferior convergence to the left of the midline at the level of the upper sacral segments. The ahaustral loop can often be identified overlapping the haustrated descending colon and the lower margin of the liver.

Gas in abscesses

The appearance of gas in abscesses is very variable. It may form a relatively large collection and on a horizontal ray film demonstrate a gas/fluid level. In these cases there is often confusion with normal bowel gas, although constant position, particularly outside and separate from normal bowel contents, will often allow a specific diagnosis to be made. Gas may, however, form small bubbles which appear similar to gas trapped within faeces. Abscesses are mass lesions and so they also displace adjacent structures.

References

Bryant L.R., Wiot J.F. & Kloecker R.J. (1963) A study of the factors affecting the incidence and duration of post-operative pneumoperitoneum. *Surg. Gynecol. Obstet.*, **117**, 145

Gammill S.L. & Nice C.M. (1972) Air fluid levels: their occurrence in normal patients and their role in the analysis of ileus. *Surgery*, **71**, 771

Grillo I.A. & Bohrer S.P. (1973) Pseudopneumoperitoneum. Linear atelectasis simulating pneumoperitoneum. *Am. Surg.*, **39**, 60

Hywel Jones J. & Chapman M. (1969) Definition of megacolon in colitis. *Gut*, **10**, 562

Menuck L. & Siemers P.T. (1976) Pneumoperitoneum. Importance of right upper quadrant features. *Am. J. Roentgenol.*, **127**, 753

Miller R.E. (1973) The technical approach to the acute abdomen. *Semin. Roentgenol.*, **8**, 267

Young W.S., Engelbrecht H.E. & Stoker A. (1978) Plain film analysis in sigmoid volvulus. *Clin. Radiol.*, **29**, 553

Further reading

Frimann-Dahl J. (1974) *Roentgen Examinations in Acute Abdominal Diseases*. Springfield, Illinois: Charles C. Thomas

McCort, J.J. (1981) *Abdominal Radiology*. Baltimore/London: Williams and Wilkins

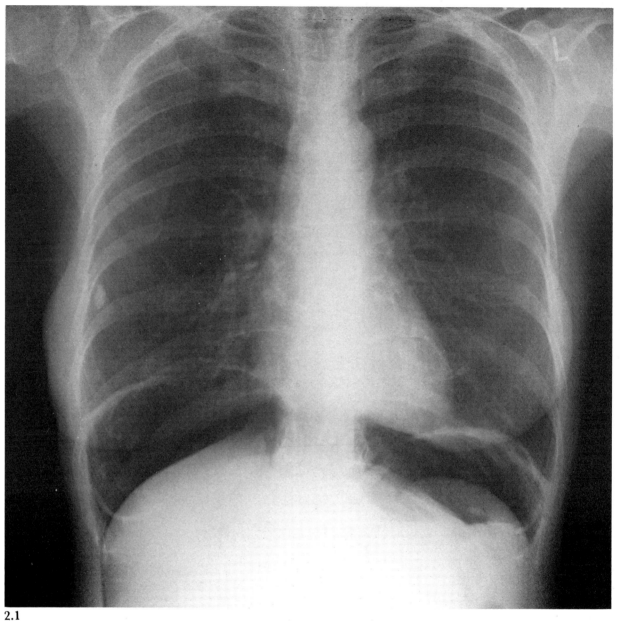

2.1
2.1 **Free intra-abdominal gas** *Erect chest radiograph*

2.2 **Free intra-abdominal gas** a *Erect chest radiograph* showing a small amount of free gas under the right hemidiaphragm. b *Right-side-up lateral decubitus abdominal radiograph* demonstrating free gas and fluid between the liver and lateral abdominal wall. The patient had been positioned for 10 minutes prior to the second radiograph being taken. The 75-year-old man with abdominal pain was shown to have a perforated gastric ulcer on subsequent laparotomy

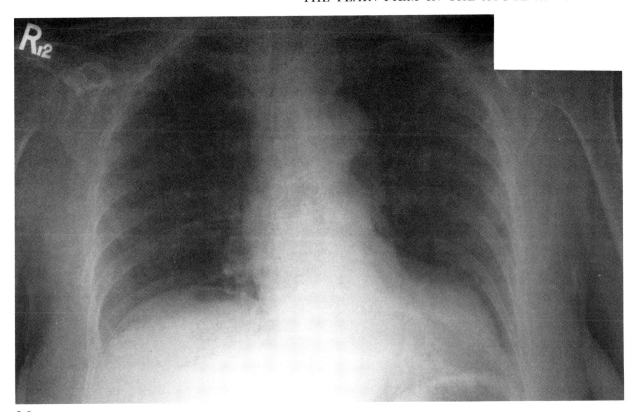

2.2a

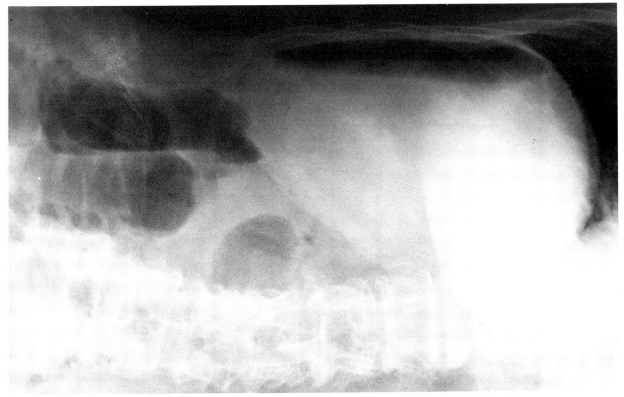

2.2b

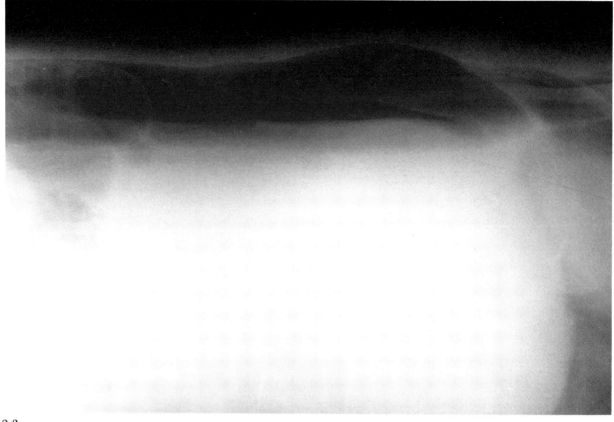

2.3

2.3 **Free intra-abdominal gas** *Supine abdominal radiograph — horizontal ray technique* demonstrating a massive amount of free intra-abdominal gas and fluid in a 47-year-old man who collapsed four days after a vagotomy and pyloroplasty for a chronic duodenal ulcer. He was so ill that erect and lateral decubitus films were not possible. At a second laparotomy, a small bowel volvulus around a mesenteric band had caused complete tearing of the suture line at the site of the pyloroplasty

2.4 **Free intra-abdominal gas** *Erect chest radiograph* demonstrating a large amount of free gas under the diaphragm in an 86-year-old woman with a perforated duodenal ulcer. There is so much free gas present that the right hemidiaphragm may be mistaken for the lesser fissure containing fluid. However, both the greater and lesser fissures can be identified separately from the diaphragm

2.5 **Curvilinear atelectasis in the left lower lobe** *Erect chest radiograph* of an 80-year-old woman who collapsed and was brought to hospital unconscious, but rapidly recovered. The linear collapse follows the curve of the diaphragm and looks very much like free gas under the diaphragm. This patient almost had a laparotomy for 'perforation'

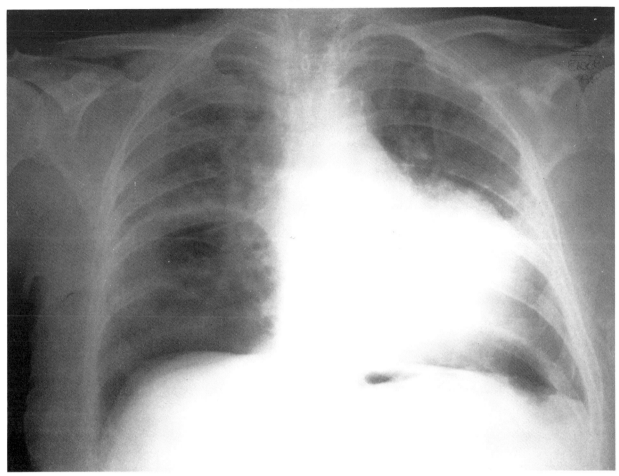

2.4

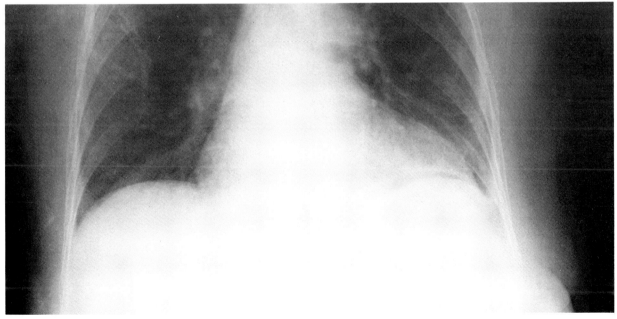

2.5

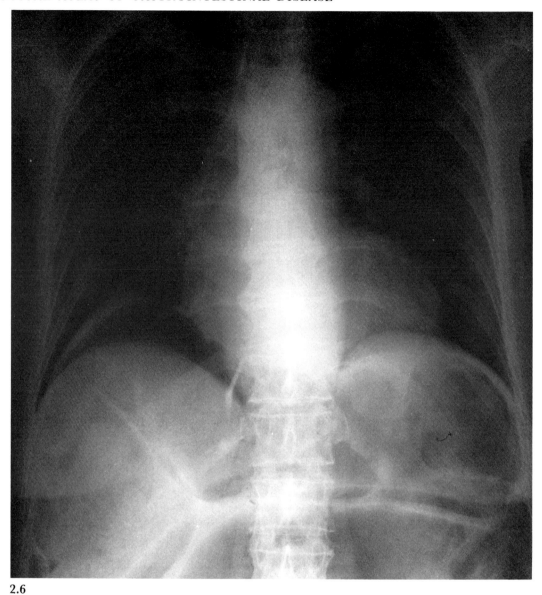

2.6

2.6 Colon interposed between the liver and diaphragm simulating free intra-abdominal gas *Erect chest radiograph* of a 63-year-old woman with abdominal pain and distension who in fact had a sigmoid volvulus

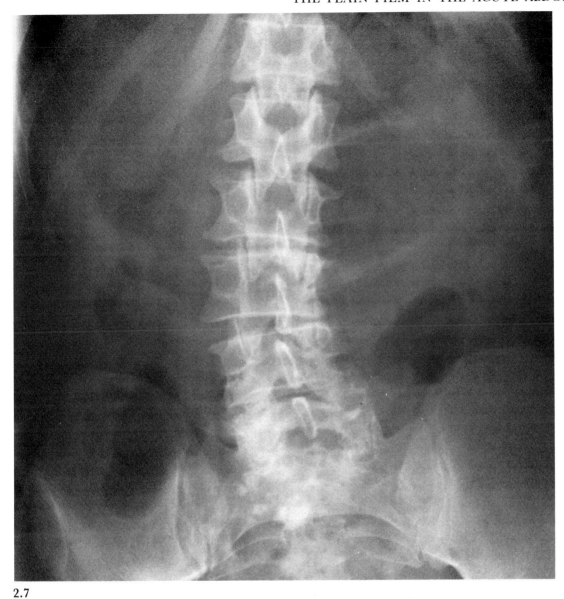

2.7

2.7 Free intra-abdominal gas *Supine abdominal radiograph* demonstrating free gas around the inferior border of the liver in a 73-year-old man with a perforated duodenal ulcer

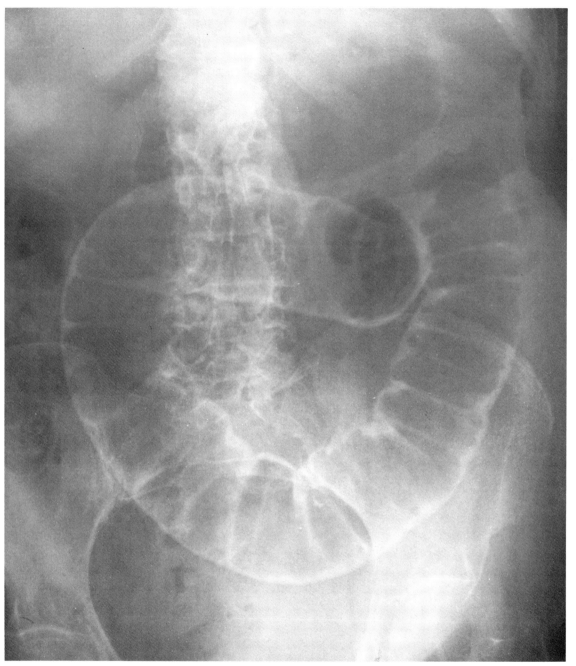

2.8

2.8 Free intra-abdominal gas *Supine abdominal radiograph* demonstrating a large amount of free gas, clearly showing gas on both sides of the bowel wall resulting in visualization of the outer wall of the bowel in an 86-year-old woman with a perforated duodenal ulcer. Same case as Figure 2.4

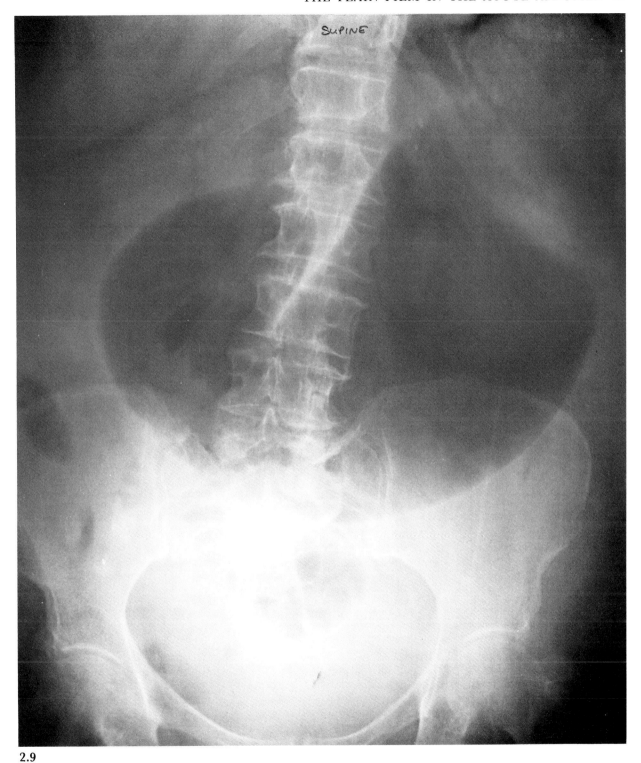

2.9

2.9 **Acute gastric dilatation** *Supine abdominal radiograph* demonstrating a distended gas-filled stomach in an 85-year-old woman with a four-day history of abdominal pain, constipation and abdominal swelling. She died before laparotomy; a perforated appendix and widespread peritonitis were found at autopsy

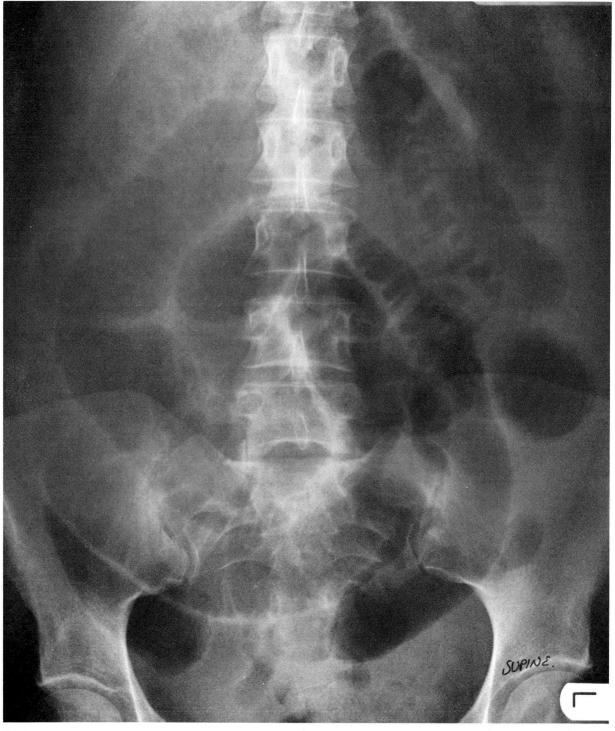

2.10a

2.10 **Small bowel obstruction** a *Supine radiograph* demonstrating multiple gas-filled dilated loops of small bowel and almost no gas in the large bowel. b *Erect abdominal radiograph* Although multiple gas/fluid levels are demonstrated in the dilated small bowel no further diagnostic information is gained. It was noticed at hysterectomy two days before that this 40-year-old woman had multiple intra-abdominal adhesions. She had persistent pain, distension and vomiting in the post-operative period

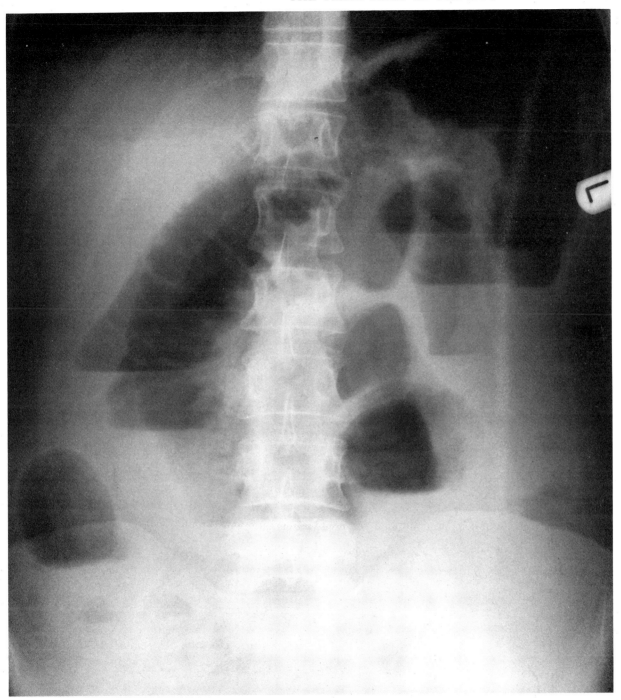

2.10b

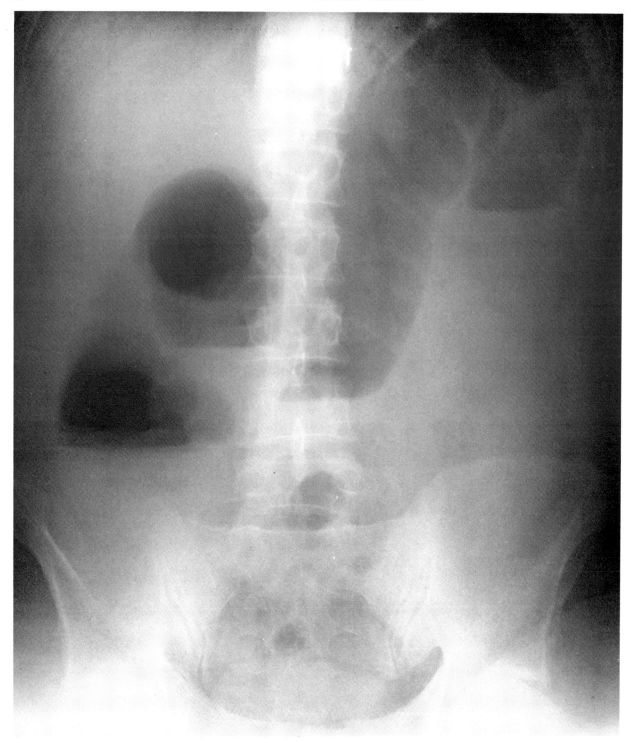

2.11a

2.11 Large bowel obstruction with a competent ileocaecal valve a *Erect abdominal radiograph* demonstrating gas/fluid levels in the dilated colon. The 55-year-old man who had received kaolin and morphine mixture for diarrhoea presented to the hospital with a three-day history of absolute constipation and abnormal distension. A hard faecal mass mixed with kaolin was found obstructing the descending colon

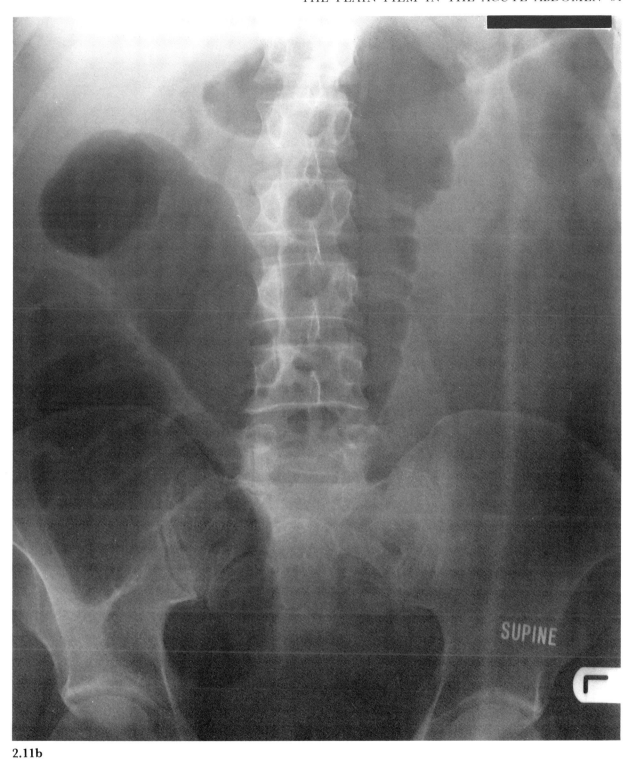

2.11b

at laparotomy. b *Supine abdominal radiograph* demonstrating gas-filled dilated colon from the caecum to the descending colon. Note the faintly calcific area just below the splenic flexure, and also the lack of small bowel filling

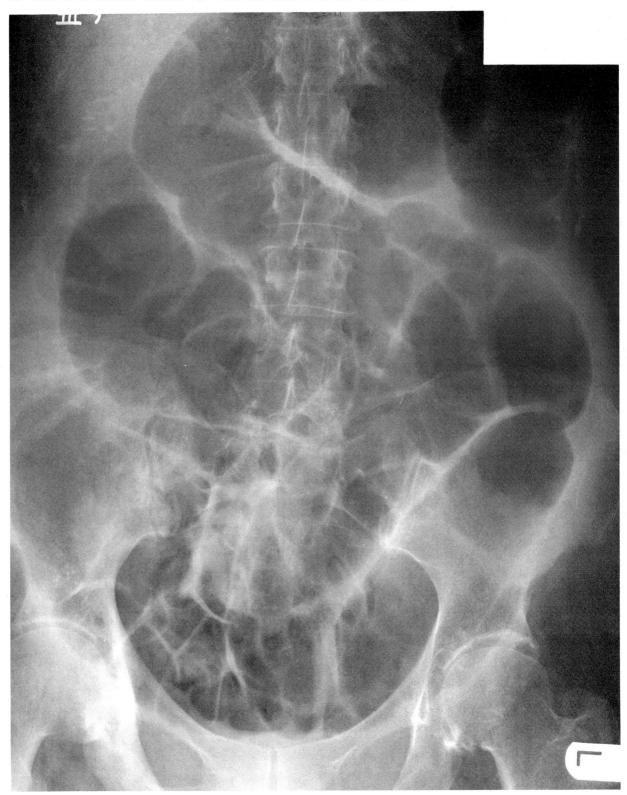

2.12a

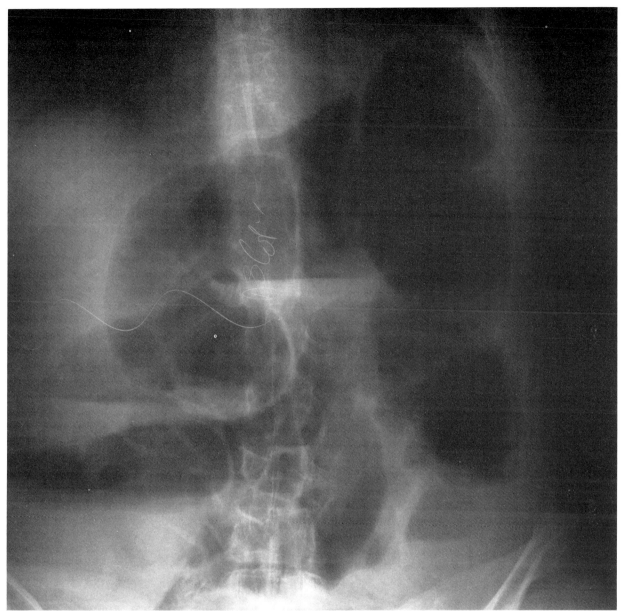

2.12b

2.12 **Large bowel obstruction with an incompetent ileocaecal valve** a *Supine radiograph* demonstrating multiple loops of dilated small bowel and large bowel as far as the sigmoid colon. b *Erect film* There are multiple air/fluid levels in the small and large bowel of a 65-year-old man with carcinoma of the rectosigmoid area who presented with colicky pain, constipation and distension over one week. Without the clinical history it would be impossible to distinguish these appearances of low large bowel obstruction from paralytic ileus. The clinical findings are essential for the correct interpretation of the plain radiograph

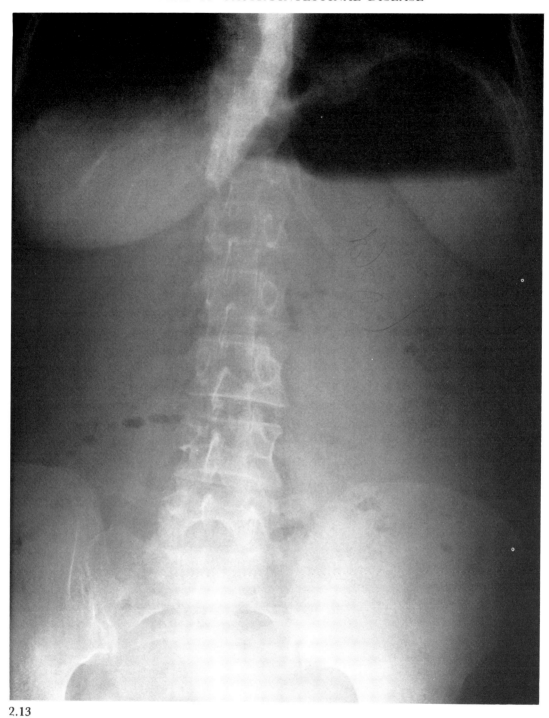

2.13

2.13 Small bowel obstruction—'string of beads' sign *Erect abdominal radiograph* showing small amounts of gas trapped between the valvulae conniventes in the dilated, mainly fluid-filled small bowel of a 12-year-old girl with diarrhoea, abdominal distension and persistent leucocytosis. At subsequent laparotomy, tuberculosis of the small bowel and peritoneum, with multiple adhesions, was found

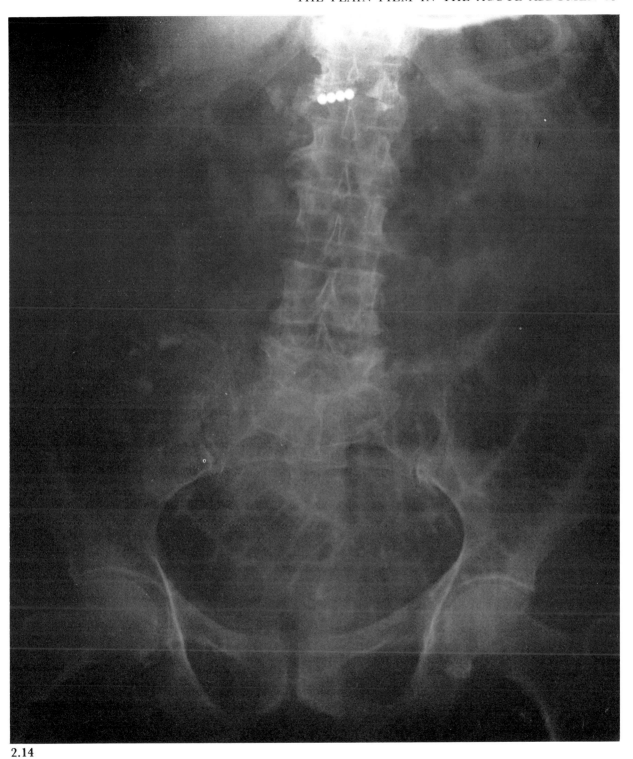

2.14

2.14 **Small bowel obstruction due to strangulated femoral hernia** *Supine abdominal radiograph* demonstrating dilated gas-filled small bowel and gas beneath the right inguinal ligament. This 82-year-old woman had small bowel obstruction due to a strangulated femoral hernia

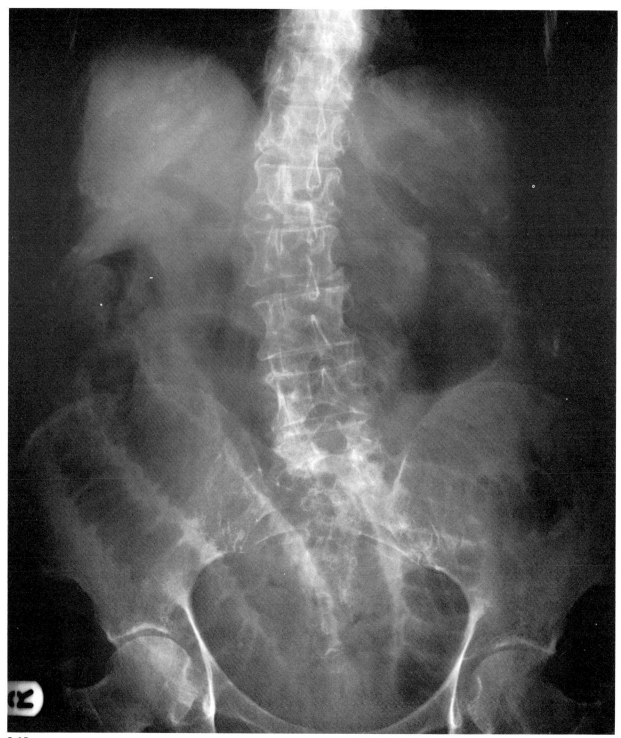

2.15

2.15 **Gallstone ileus** *Supine abdominal radiograph* demonstrating gas-filled dilated small bowel and gas in dilated bile ducts in a 78-year-old woman with several days' abdominal distension and vomiting. At laparotomy a gallstone ileus was found

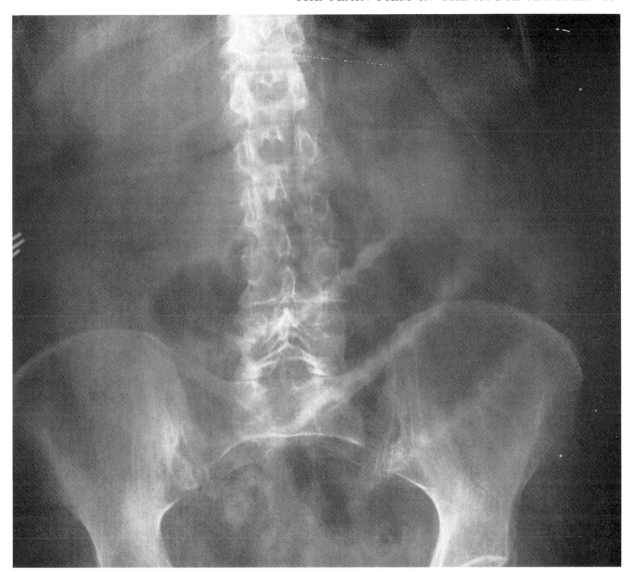

2.16

2.16 **Gallstone ileus** *Supine abdominal radiograph* demonstrating dilated gas-filled loops of small bowel and a slightly calcified gallstone overlying the right side of the sacrum in a 73-year-old woman with several days' abdominal pain and vomiting

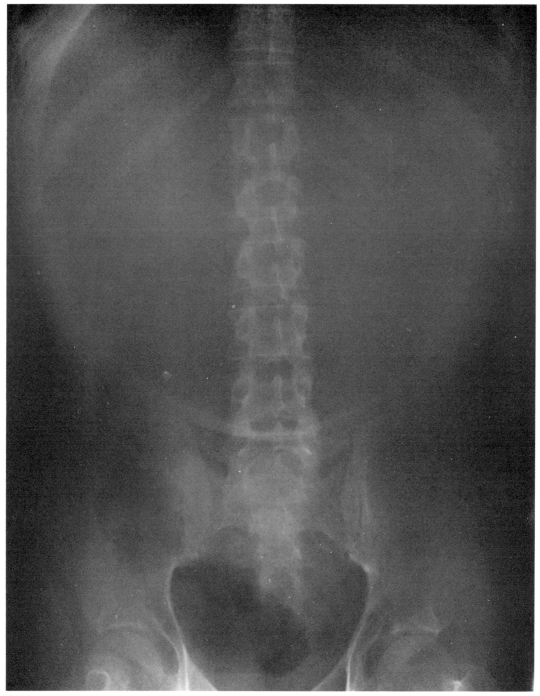

2.17

2.17 **Gastric volvulus** *Supine radiograph* showing a massively dilated gas-filled stomach in a 35-year-old patient with Down's syndrome who presented with severe pain

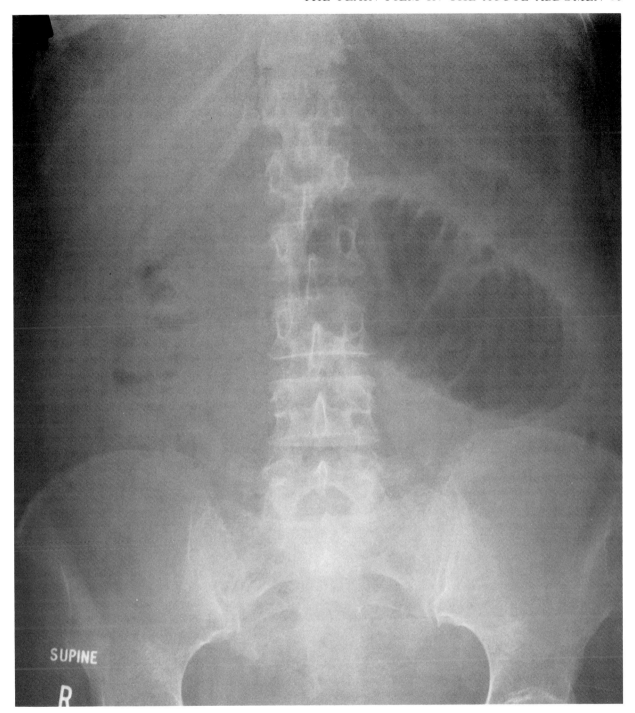

SUPINE

R

2.18

2.18 Small bowel volvulus *Supine radiograph* showing a loop of massively dilated small bowel in a 55-year-old woman who had a partial gastrectomy with a roux-en-y gastroenterostomy for a chronic duodenal ulcer. She developed severe pain one week post-operatively. The efferent loop had undergone an organoaxial volvulus.

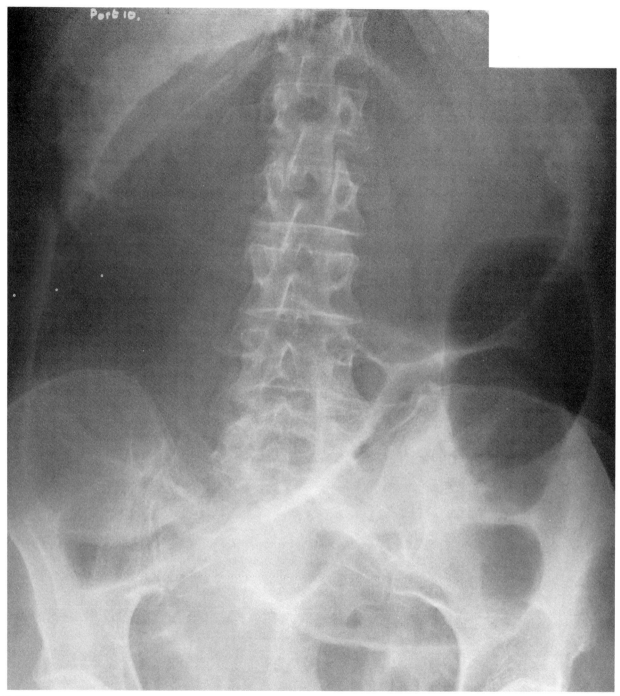

2.19a

2.19 **Caecal volvulus** a *Supine radiograph* showing a massively dilated caecum pointing up towards the left hypochondrium and many dilated loops of small bowel in a 66-year-old chronic schizophrenic with pain and vomiting for six days. b *Erect film* showing fluid level in the caecum

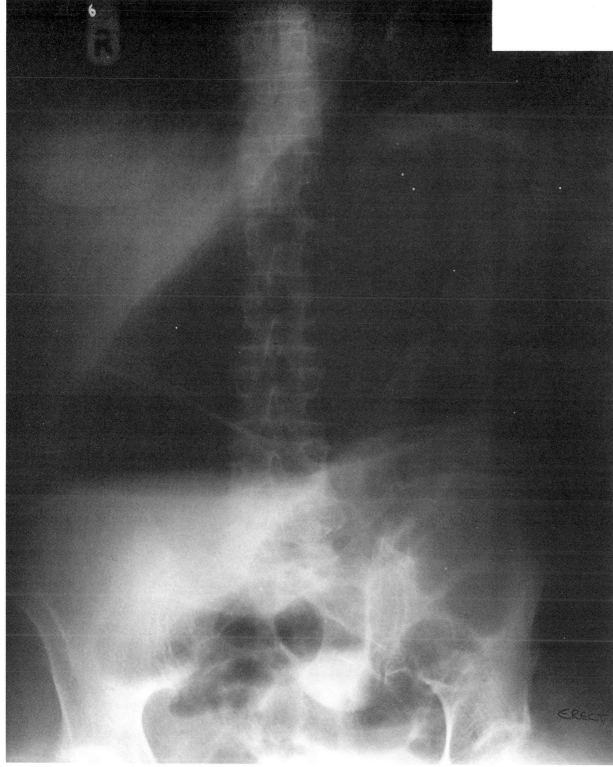

2.19b

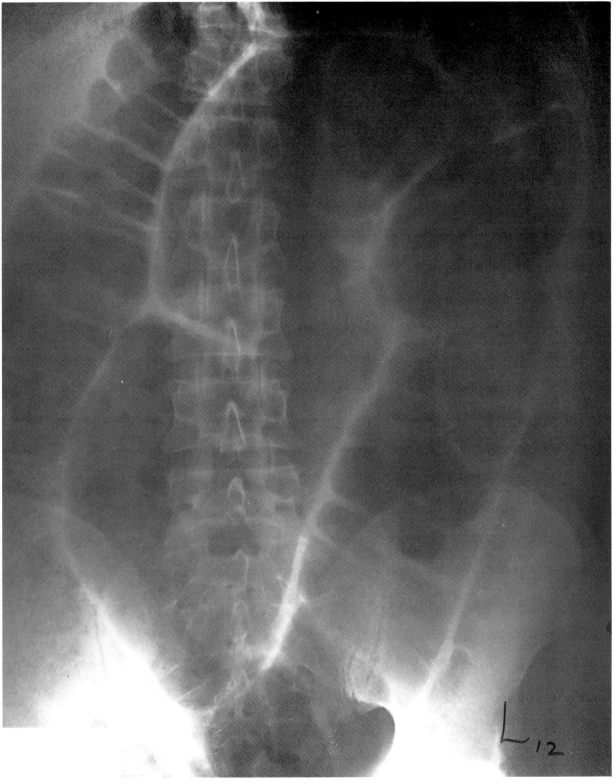

2.20

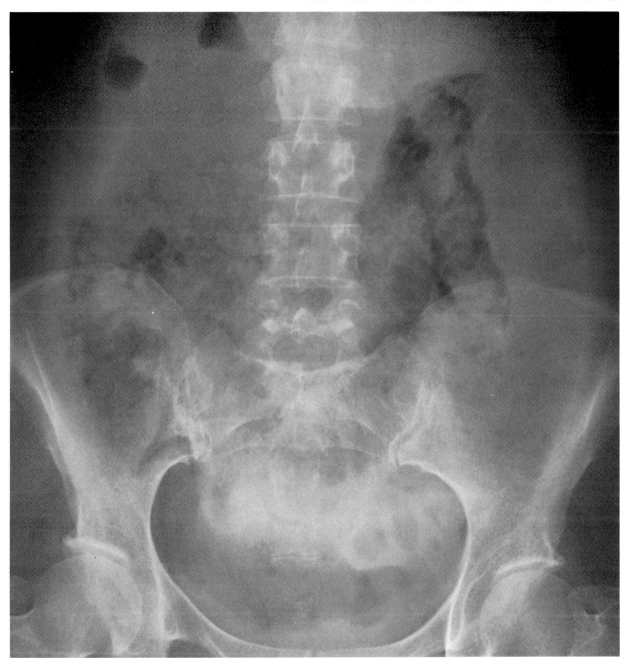

2.21

2.20 **Sigmoid volvulus** *Supine film* shows a gas-filled dilated loop of sigmoid colon ascending from the pelvis; the remainder of the large bowel is also gas-filled and distended. The 42-year-old man had colicky abdominal pain for three days

2.21 **Intramural gas** *Supine radiograph* showing extensive gas within the wall of the small bowel. In addition, note the free gas around the subhepatic region. This 52-year-old woman had total gangrene of the small bowel and perforation following metastatic spread of a primary small bowel carcinoma to involve the root of the mesentery and the superior mesenteric artery

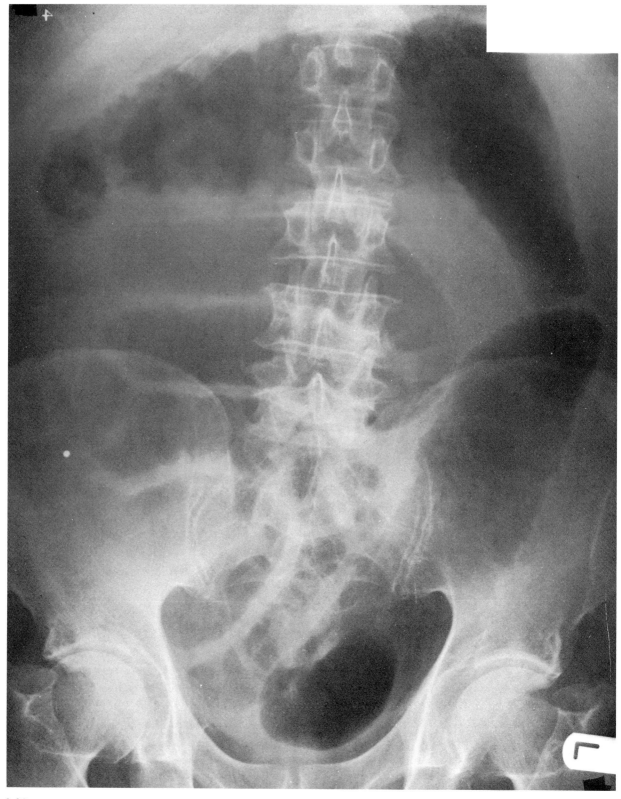

2.22a

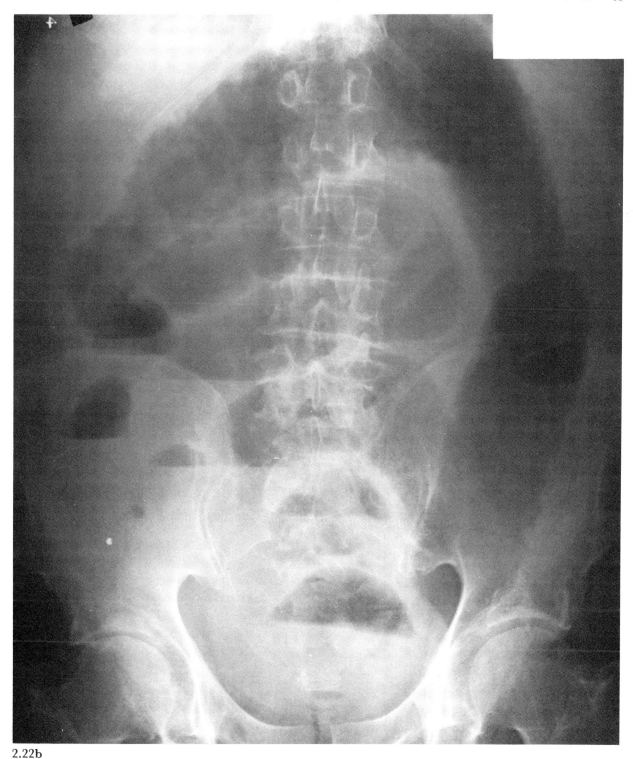

2.22b

2.22 **Toxic megacolon** a *Supine film* shows a gas-filled dilated colon with an abnormal mucosal pattern, loss of haustration and pseudopolyp formation particularly in the transverse colon. Note also the dilated small bowel. b *Erect film* demonstrating gas/fluid levels in dilated large and small bowel. The 64-year-old woman had exacerbation of ulcerative colitis

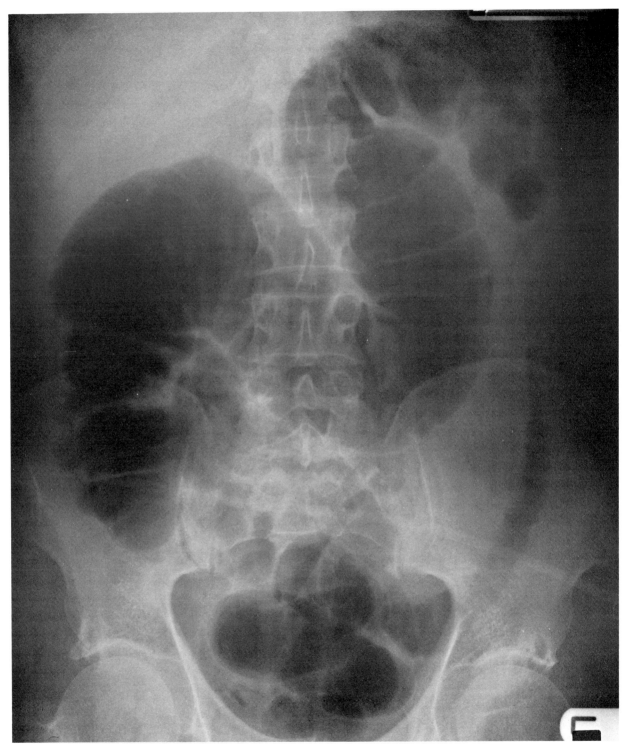

2.23a

2.23 **Ischaemic colitis** a *Supine radiograph* showing the abnormal mucosal pattern and the thick-walled descending colon in a 62-year-old man with sudden onset of pain followed by bloody diarrhoea. The colon proximal to the ischaemic area is dilated but has a normal haustral pattern. The ischaemic area is acting as an area of functional obstruction. b *Barium enema examination* shows the abnormal mucosal pattern caused by submucosal oedema and haemorrhage

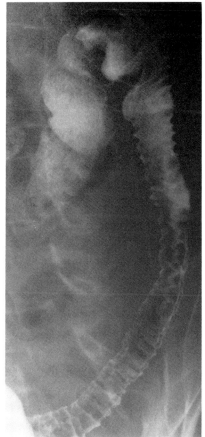

2.23b

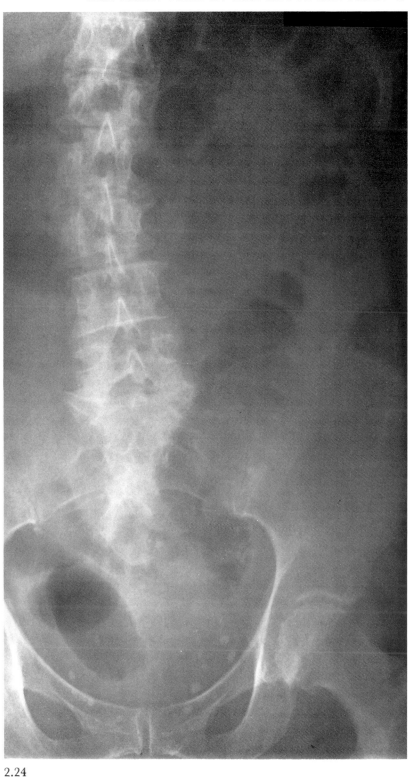
2.24

2.24 **Pericolic abscess due to perforated diverticular disease** *Supine radiograph* shows the gas-filled normally haustrated descending colon displaced medially by a large mass which is predominantly gas-filled. The abscess was not suspected clinically in this 81-year-old woman but was confirmed on laparotomy

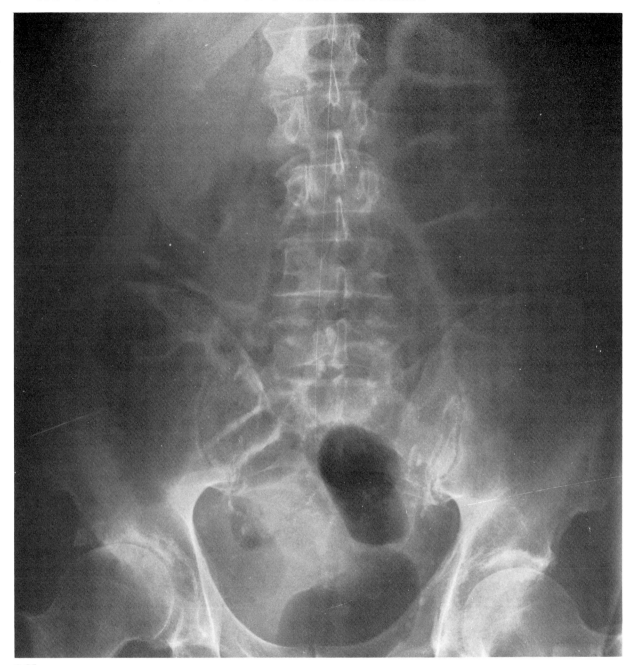

2.25a

2.25 **Appendix abscess** a *Supine radiograph* demonstrating a large soft tissue mass in the right pelvis which is displacing the pelvic colon to the left and indenting the caecal pole. In the centre of the mass there is a collection of gas. b *Erect film* confirms the soft tissue mass containing a gas/fluid level and also demonstrates a fluid level in the caecum—the latter is a common *normal* finding. The 77-year-old man had diarrhoea and right iliac fossa pain for one week.

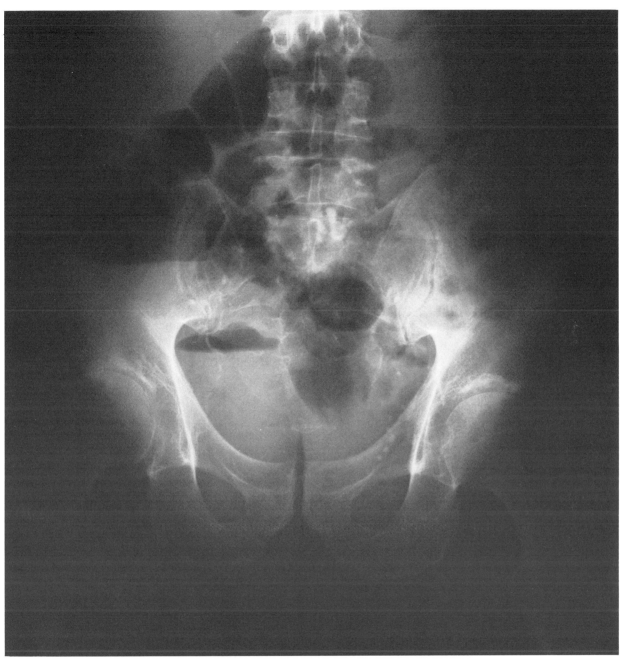

2.25b

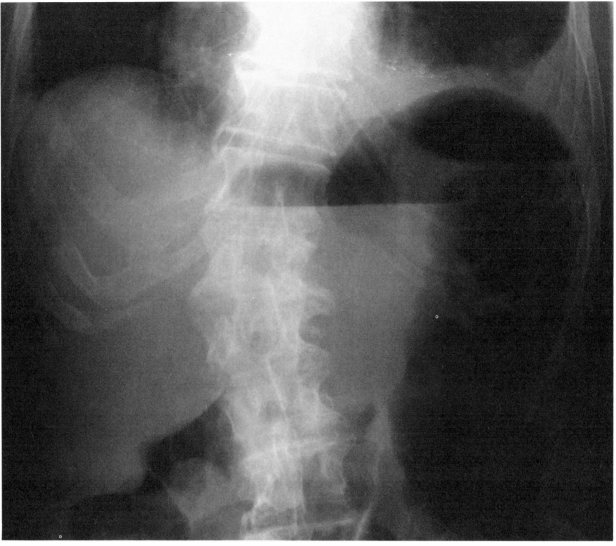

2.26

2.26 **Subphrenic abscess** *Erect film* shows gas/fluid levels at two heights—separate from the colon and anatomically incorrect for the stomach. Note also the left-sided pleural effusion. The 73-year-old man was sent for a barium meal with a three-week history of anorexia, vomiting and weight loss. The subphrenic abscess was confirmed at laparotomy and was due to a perforated gastric ulcer

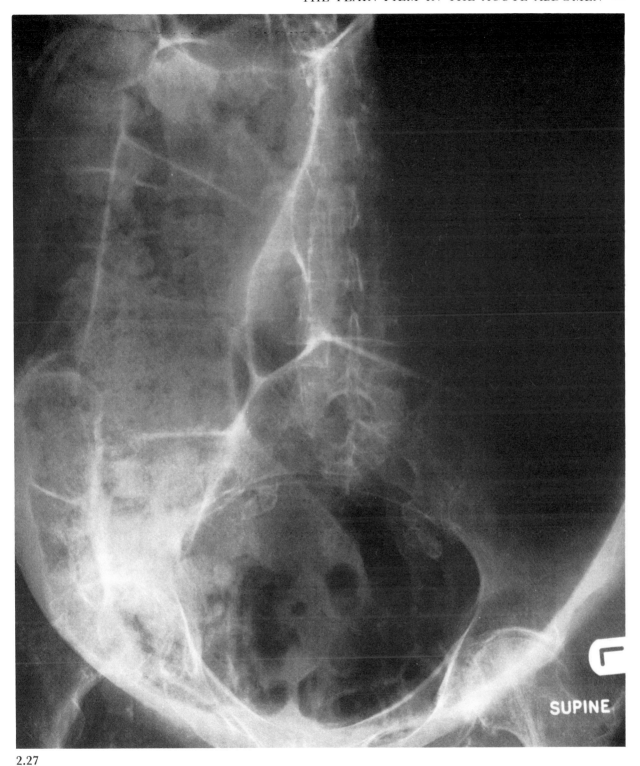

2.27

2.27 **Pseudo-obstruction** *Supine radiograph* demonstrating massive gaseous distension of the colon— the descending colon measures 21 cm in diameter—and is indistinguishable from chronic low large bowel obstruction on plain films. Barium enema examination showed no obstructing lesion in the 93-year-old woman with progressive abdominal distension, pain and constipation

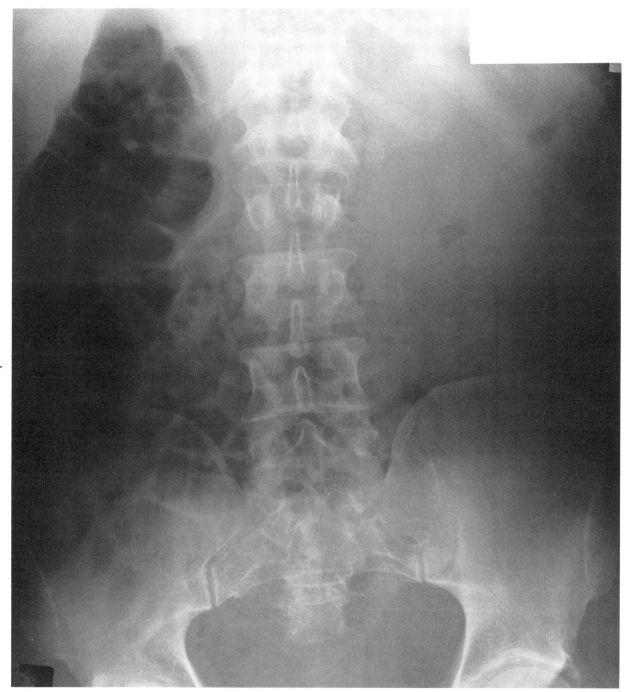

2.28a

2.28 **Large bowel ileus secondary to a urinoma** a *Supine radiograph* shows a large soft tissue mass in the left hypochondrium and lack of gas in the left half of the colon. The right side of the colon is gas-filled and slightly dilated. b *Intravenous urogram—10-minute film* There is extravasation of contrast from the left renal pelvis down the psoas and retroperitoneally. This is an example of spontaneous rupture of a renal pelvis in a 52-year-old man with pelviureteric junction obstruction. The retroperitoneal collection of urine (urinoma) has caused a secondary ileus of the colon. The patient presented with symptoms indistinguishable from large bowel obstruction—abdominal pain, distension and constipation

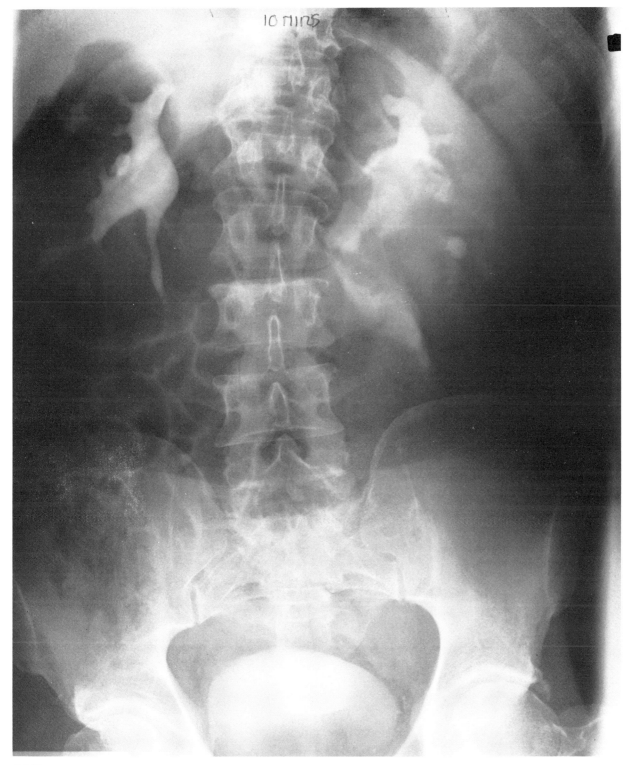

2.28b

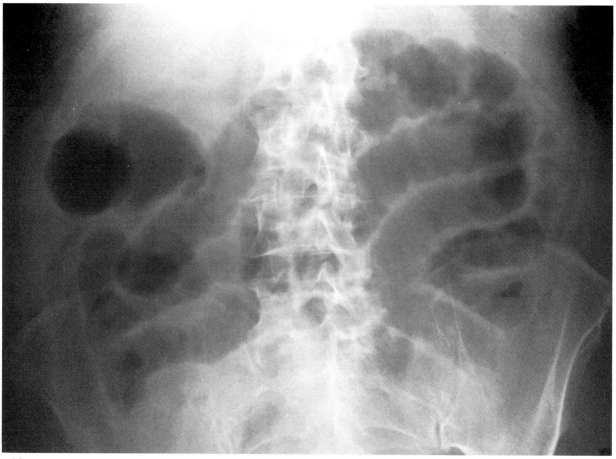

2.29

2.29 **Mesenteric infarction** *Supine radiograph* showing many loops of a gas-filled but not particularly dilated small bowel in a 73-year-old woman with atrial fibrillation who developed sudden severe abdominal pain

Duplications

Duplications are spherical or elongated structures attached to the gastrointestinal tract which are congenital in origin (Borrie 1961). They possess a smooth-muscle coat and are lined with mucous membrane. They may communicate with the gastrointestinal tract, forming diverticula or large duplications. The majority, however, do not communicate with the lumen but form cysts. Symptoms develop as a result of obstruction of the adjacent gastrointestinal tract, or pain from fluid distension, bleeding or perforation (Borrie 1961).

Oesophageal duplications are more common and larger on the right side and rarely communicate with the oesophagus. Radiologically they are shown as space-occupying lesions in the posterior mediastinum, related to the oesophagus. Communicating duplications may appear as cavitating lesions similar to large ulcers.

Gastric duplications occur but rarely. Diverticula are the commonest anomaly in the stomach. They are seen mainly on the posterior aspect of the upper end of the lesser curve and only occasionally cause symptoms. The characteristic location of diverticula, mucosal folds seen passing into the diverticulum, the absence of oedema and radiating folds are all factors that distinguish them from peptic ulcers.

Duplications occur most frequently in the small intestine, including the duodenum, where they may cause obstruction, perforation of the intestine or intussusception. Heterotopia, particularly when the ectopic mucosa is gastric in type, may produce ulceration with pain and bleeding (Anderson *et al.* 1962). A communicating duplication, seen as a diverticulum, may be an incidental finding during barium studies. Duplications of the colon are often double-barrelled and may extend the entire length of the colon and rectum (Anderson *et al.* 1962).

Pyloric stenosis

The majority of cases of hypertrophic pyloric stenosis present in infancy. Pyloric stenosis in adults may represent a delayed manifestation of the infantile disease, although the number of such cases is small (Lumsden & Truelove 1958). Radiologically the pyloric end of the gastric antrum is elongated and narrowed and there may be excessive fluid in the stomach.

Pancreatic rests

Aberrant pancreatic tissue may involve the gastric antrum of the stomach and can cause dyspepsia, bleeding or obstruction. It is often an incidental finding on barium studies and is shown on the greater curve of the prepyloric gastric antrum as a small polypoid lesion with a central umbilicated area containing barium.

3 Developmental Anomalies

Musosal diaphragm

A congenital mucosal diaphragm of the gastric antrum and pylorus may only produce symptoms late in life. The classic symptoms are epigastric discomfort or pain after eating which is relieved by vomiting. Diagnosis was made on X-ray in nine of the thirteen patients reviewed by Banks *et al.* (1967). The diaphragm was described as a linear, knife-like defect in the antrum, present on all projections.

Duodenocolic fistula

Duodenocolic fistula of developmental origin may present late in life. Three such patients, aged between 47 and 51 years, were reported by Torrance & Jones (1972). Diarrhoea and weight loss are the usual presenting features. The communication occurs between the third part of the duodenum and the transverse colon and is easily demonstrated by a barium study of the upper gastrointestinal tract or colon.

Meckel's diverticulum

Meckel's diverticulum, the persisting proximal portion of the vitellointestinal duct, is present in 1–4 per cent of individuals (Morson & Dawson 1979). It lies on the antimesenteric border of the ileum within 91 cm of the ileocaecal valve and the size varies from 1 to 5 cm in diameter (DeBartolo & van Heerden 1976). The diverticulum is usually lined with normal small intestinal mucosa but heterotopic gastric mucosa may be present and cause peptic ulceration. Most symptomatic diverticula present as a result of gastrointestinal bleeding, manifested as either anaemia from chronic blood loss or episodes of melaena. Inflammation can also occur and lead to abdominal pain, adhesions and sometimes obstruction.

Meckel's diverticulum is shown on a barium study as a blind sac attached to the antimesenteric border of the distal small intestine (Maglinte *et al.* 1980). Angiography and radionuclide studies are other techniques used to detect Meckel's diverticulum containing heterotopic gastric mucosa.

Anomalies of rotation

Anomalies of rotation frequently result in volvulus or intestinal obstruction. Non-rotation, malrotation, reversed rotation and paraduodenal hernia result from faulty rotation during the second stage in embryonic life (Wang & Welch 1963). Non-rotation is uncommon—the duodenum descends down on the right side of the superior mesenteric artery in direct continuity with the small intestine, which is located on the right side of the abdominal cavity. The colon is located in the left side of the abdominal cavity and the terminal ileum crosses the mid-line to enter the caecum.

Malrotation is the most commonly encountered and occurs when the midgut does not complete the entire rotation in an anticlockwise direction. The caecum may become arrested—most commonly in the subhepatic region, but also in front of the mesenteric vessels or at the splenic level (Wang & Welch 1963). Reversed rotation is rare and occurs when there is rotation in a reversed direction, i.e. clockwise. The caecum and transverse colon pass through the root of the mesentery behind the superior mesenteric artery and the duodenum is in front. Paraduodenal hernia is a rare congenital anomaly of intestinal rotation.

Anomalies arising from the third stage of rotation may cause the small intestine to have a mesentery with a long and narrow pedicle and deficient fixation. The second and third parts of the duodenum may be free and mobile.

Situs inversus

Reversal in position of the abdominal organs is termed situs inversus. The thoracic as well as the abdominal organs are involved in complete situs inversus, whereas if the abdominal organs only are reversed it is incomplete situs inversus.

Tumour-like malformations

Tumours such as hamartomas, neurofibromas and haemangiomas are developmental in origin, but as they resemble other gastrointestinal tract tumours they are included in the differential diagnosis and are illustrated in the appropriate sections of the book.

Hirschsprung's disease (aganglionic megacolon)

In this condition there is marked dilation of the colon proximal to a relatively narrowed segment of aganglionic intestine (Davidson 1978). The aganglionic segment extends proximally from the internal anal sphincter for varying lengths. The extent of the aganglionic segment is determined by barium enema examination. It is performed without colon preparation and the infusion is stopped as soon as barium begins to outline the dilated segment.

References

Anderson M.C., Silberman W.W. & Shields T.W. (1962) Duplications of the alimentary tract. *Arch. Surg.*, **85**, 94

Banks P.A., Waye J.D., Waitman A.M. & Cornell A. (1967) Mucosal diaphragm of the gastric antrum. *Gastroenterology*, **52**, 1003

Borrie J. (1961) Duplication of the oesophagus. *Br. J. Surg.*, **48**, 611

Davidson M. (1978) Megacolon in children. In *Gastrointestinal Disease* (Eds. Sleisenger M.H. & Fordtran J.S.). Philadelphia: W.B. Saunders

DeBartolo H.M. & van Heerden J.A. (1976) Meckel's diverticulum. *Ann. Surg.*, **183**, 30

Lumsden K. & Truelove S.C. (1958) Primary hypertrophic pyloric stenosis in the adult. *Br. J. Radiol.*, **31**, 261

Lumsden K. & Truelove S.C. (1965) *Radiology of the Digestive System*. Oxford: Blackwell Scientific Publications

Maglinte D.D., Elmore M.F., Isenberg M. & Dolan P.A. (1980) Meckel diverticulum: radiologic demonstration by enteroclysis. *Am. J. Roetgenol.*, **134**, 925

Morson B.C. & Dawson I.M.P. (1979) *Gastrointestinal Pathology*. Oxford: Blackwell Scientific Publications

Torrance B. & Jones C. (1972) Three cases of spontaneous duodeno-colic fistula. *Gut*, **13**, 627

Wang C.-A. & Welch C.E. (1963) Anomalies of intestinal rotation in adolescents and adults. *Surgery*, **54**, 839

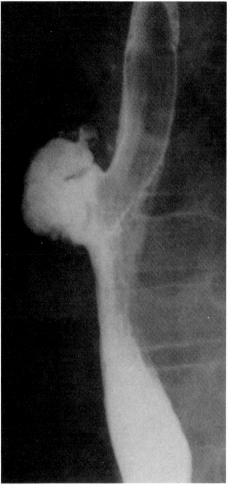

3.1

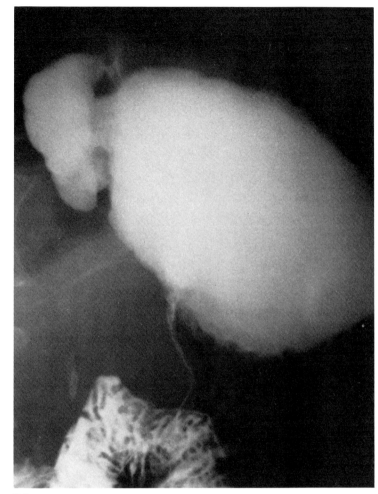

3.3

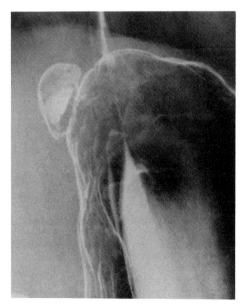

3.2

3.1 **Oesophageal duplication** A large slightly irregular cavity on the right side of the mid oesophagus is outlined with barium. The patient, a 13-year-old girl, was admitted to hospital with haematemesis. The lesion was resected and on examination proved to be a duplication cyst

3.2 **Gastric diverticulum** A moderate-sized diverticulum is seen on the posterior aspect of the upper end of the lesser curve of the stomach

3.3 **Gastric diverticulum** A large barium-filled diverticulum is seen passing posteriorly from the upper end of the lesser curve of the stomach in a patient whose symptoms were not caused by the diverticulum

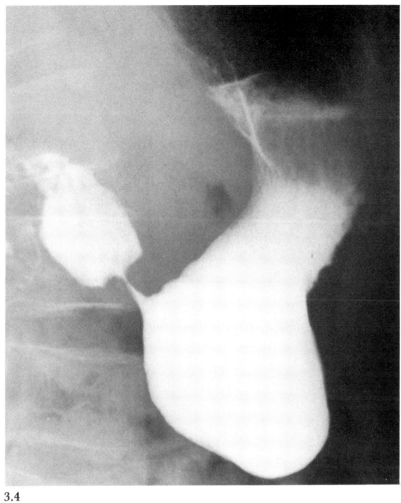

3.4

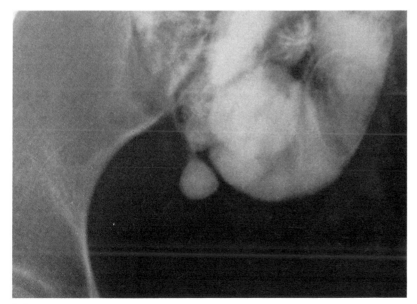

3.5

3.4 **Hypertrophic pyloric stenosis** in an adult (Lumsden & Truelove, 1965)

3.5 **Meckel's diverticulum** A small diverticulum is seen on the antimesenteric border of the distal ileum. This was an incidental finding in a patient who presented with right-sided abdominal pain. The Meckel's diverticulum and adjacent ileum were freely mobile

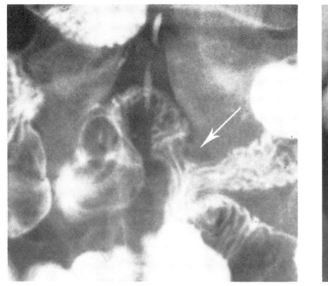

3.6

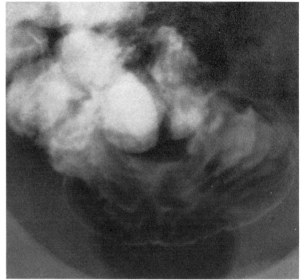

3.7

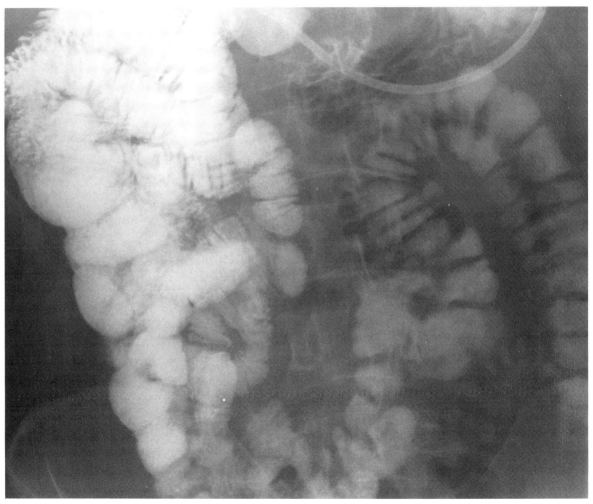

3.8

3.6 **Meckel's diverticulum** There is a moderate-sized ileal diverticulum containing a polypoid filling defect. The triradiate fold pattern (arrow) is characteristic of Meckel's diverticulum. The patient, a 36-year-old man, presented with abdominal pain and anaemia; a Meckel's diverticulum was confirmed at operation. Histological examination showed that the polypoid mass represented mucus-secreting gastric epithelium (Maglinte *et al.* 1980)

3.7 **Meckel's diverticulum** A large diverticulum of the distal ileum is seen. The mucosal pattern in the diverticulum is similar to gastric mucosa, giving the diverticulum the appearance of a small stomach. The 29-year-old man was investigated for anaemia. The presence of a large Meckel's diverticulum containing heterotopic gastric mucosa was confirmed at operation

3.8 **Non-rotation** The duodenum, jejunum and ileum are on the right side of the abdomen. The colon is located on the left side and the terminal ileum is seen crossing the midline to enter the caecum

3.9 **Hirschsprung's disease** A short narrowed aganglionic segment of rectum is seen with dilatation of the colon proximal to the narrowed segment

3.10 **Hirschsprung's disease** a The aganglionic segment of distal sigmoid colon and rectum is of normal calibre. b The more proximal colon is dilated and contains a large amount of faecal material

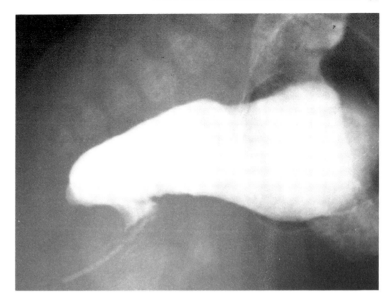

3.9

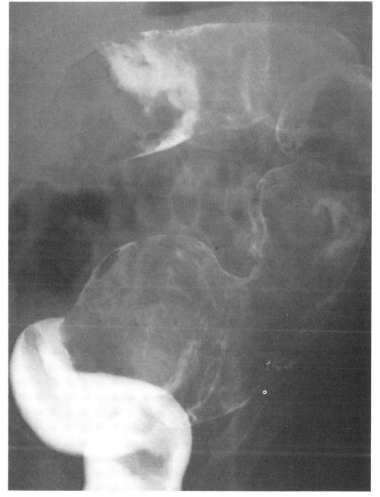

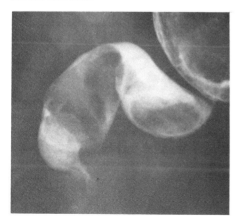

3.10a

3.10b

Hiatal hernia and oesophagitis

The term hiatal hernia refers to the presence in the chest, above the diaphragm, of a pouch of stomach that has passed through the normal oesophageal hiatus (Spiro 1977). Hiatal hernias may be small or large and are classified as sliding and rolling types. The sliding hernia occurs when the lower end of the oesophagus, oesophagogastric junction and cardia of the stomach slide upwards through the hiatus. It may be small with only a small part of the stomach passing into the chest, or large when nearly all the stomach herniates. The rolling (paraoesophageal) type of hernia is uncommon; the stomach passes upwards through the hiatus to lie beside the oesophagus while the lower end of the oesophagus and the oesophagogastric junction remain below the diaphragm. Mixed sliding and rolling hernias sometimes occur. Many hiatal hernias, even large ones, are asymptomatic. Symptoms develop from complications such as ulceration, oesophagitis, oesophageal stricture, bleeding or incarceration.

Oesophagitis is a result of gastric acid refluxing into the oesophagus from the stomach. Acid reflux is common in patients with sliding hiatal hernias but it can also occur in the absence of hiatal hernia. Chest pain, often described as heartburn, is the main symptom of oesophagitis. The double-contrast barium study is superior to the single-contrast examination for demonstrating the changes caused by peptic oesophagitis. The signs are thickening of the folds, granularity, plaques, ulceration and luminal narrowing, mostly in the lower oesophagus (Kressel *et al.* 1981). The folds are considered abnormal if they are greater than 2 mm in an oesophagus that is distended more than 2 cm. Ill-defined lucencies, 1–2 mm in size in the distended oesophagus, are defined as granularity, and discrete 2–3 mm elevations of the oesophageal mucosa are plaques.

Benign strictures

Narrowing of the lumen of the oesophagus with stricture formation occurs as a complication of a number of conditions. Peptic strictures resulting from reflux oesophagitis are the most common benign strictures. A sliding type hiatal hernia is frequently seen in association with oesophageal strictures. Patients usually present with dysphagia. Benign strictures are usually found at the lower end of the oesophagus and show symmetrical narrowing often with smooth margins, although the stricture may have an irregular margin suggestive of malignancy. It may be impossible to differentiate a benign stricture from carcinoma, and endoscopic biopsies should always be obtained to confirm the diagnosis.

The lower margins of the narrowed segment of oesophagus should be clearly demonstrated on barium studies. If the patient swallows barium in the horizontal position at double-contrast barium examination, a large volume of gas refluxes from the stomach causing distension of the cardia and lower oesophagus. This allows the lower margin to be clearly shown and the length

4 The Oesophagus

of the stricture assessed. The lower end of a stricture can also be shown clearly if the patient swallows the barium in the Trendelenburg position.

A combination of columnar epithelium lining the lower oesophagus, stricture, oesophageal ulcer and hiatal hernia was described by Barrett in 1950—the columnar-lined oesophagus or Barrett's syndrome. Originally it was thought that some cases were developmental in origin but it is now considered to be an acquired condition caused by gastro-oesophageal reflux. A ring-like constriction in the lower oesophagus is sometimes found in patients with dysphagia. This lower oesophageal ring (Schatzki's ring) is probably due to a fold of mucosa located at or above the squamocolumnar junction (Goyal et al. 1971).

Prolonged nasogastric intubation may result in the development of oesophageal strictures. The first symptoms of stricture formation become evident weeks or months later (Banfield & Hurwitz 1974). Post-intubation strictures are seen as long smooth narrowing in the distal third of the oesophagus.

Oesophageal strictures can occur as a late complication following ingestion of acid and alkaline caustic material. Such strictures are frequently long, involving the upper and mid oesophagus and sometimes the lower oesophagus. Strictures of the mid oesophagus may develop as a result of potassium therapy in cases of left atrial enlargement—usually patients who have undergone cardiac surgery for rheumatic heart disease. A small percentage of patients develop an oesophageal stricture within the field of previous radiation therapy (Rogers & Goldstein 1977). Radiation strictures have a benign appearance with tapered margins and relatively smooth mucosal surfaces.

Oesophageal tuberculosis is uncommon but can result in the formation of a benign stricture. Tuberculous strictures of the oesophagus are usually irregular, often with ulceration and sinus track formation (Schneider 1976). Strictures of the oesophagus as a result of involvement with Crohn's disease are rare (Dyer et al. 1969).

Tumours

Benign tumours of the oesophagus are uncommon—leiomyomas are the type most frequently encountered. They are seen radiologically as smooth indentations of the mid or lower third of the oesophagus. Other benign tumours occasionally seen include hamartomas, adenomas and lipomas.

The majority of malignant oesophageal tumours are squamous cell carcinomas, but a significant number of adenocarcinomas occur in the lower third, while other types such as carcinosarcomas and melanomas are seen occasionally (Morson & Dawson 1979). In the upper oesophagus post-cricoid carcinoma is common in women and is often associated with sideropenic dysphagia (Patterson–Kelly or Plummer–Vinson syndrome). Heavy smoking and excessive alcohol consumption increase the risk of developing carcinoma of the oesophagus (Wynder & Bross 1961). The most frequent clinical presentation is dysphagia. Acute gastrointestinal bleeding or pulmonary symptoms from aspiration are other modes of presentation. Carcinomas of the oesophagus are shown radiologically as infiltrating, polypoid or ulcerating lesions.

Extrinsic compression

Narrowing of the oesophagus may result from compression by an adjacent mass such as carcinoma or tuberculosis of the mediastinum. When a retrosternal goitre causes compression with marked narrowing of the oesophagus the possibility of a thyroid carcinoma should always be considered.

Diverticula

Most oesophageal diverticula are acquired; they are classified as pulsion diverticula and traction diverticula. Pulsion diverticula are high-pressure phenomena developing within or above an area of diffuse spasm, or above a hyperactive sphincter (Cross et al. 1961). They are frequently found in association with other oesophageal disorders. Pharyngo-oesophageal (Zenker's) diverticulum results from herniation of hypopharangeal mucosa and submucosa through a point of weakness in the fibres of oblique and circular muscles (Shirazi et al. 1977). It develops slowly and increases in size over a period of years. Dysphagia is the usual presenting symptom in patients with Zenker's diverticula. Regurgitation of food or recurrent respiratory infections due to aspiration are other symptoms. Small Zenker's diverticula are often an incidental finding during barium studies.

Epiphrenic diverticula are a type of pulsion diverticula seen occasionally. They occur mostly on the right side just above the oesophagogastric junction and are usually asymptomatic. Adhesions to tuberculous mediastinal lymph glands can cause traction diverticula to develop. There is scarring and contraction of the inflamed tissue and the wall of the oesophagus is drawn out in a tent-like fashion.

Intramural pseudodiverticulosis of the oesophagus is a rare condition characterized by multiple small flask-like out-pouchings in the oesophageal wall (Cho *et al.* 1981). Patients present with dysphagia and there is evidence of oesophagitis in a high percentage of cases.

Oesophageal varices

When the portal system is obstructed a remarkable collateral circulation develops to carry portal blood into the systemic veins (Sherlock 1981). Oesophageal and gastric varices develop as part of this collateral circulation. Hepatic cirrhosis is the most common cause of portal hypertension. The earliest radiological finding is localized thickening of the mucosal folds, with a wavy appearance of the borders and slight dilatation of the oesophagus (Zaino & Beneventano 1977). In more advanced cases the varices are seen as multiple round filling defects in the lower third of the oesophagus. With further progression of the disease varices may be present in the middle and upper third of the oesophagus. 'Downhill' varices are only seen in the upper third of the oesophagus, usually in association with superior vena caval obstruction or mediastinal fibrosis.

Oesophageal varices can also be demonstrated at transplenic portal venography, on the venous phase of selective coeliac angiography and by transhepatic portography (Lunderquist & Vang 1974). The latter technique is usually performed as the preliminary part of a therapeutic procedure to sclerose the varices.

Post-cricoid webs

The condition characterized by dysphagia due to post-cricoid webs, glossitis, koilonychia and iron deficiency anaemia is known as sideropenic dysphagia, the Plummer–Vinson syndrome, or the Patterson–Kelly syndrome. Most patients who develop a post-cricoid web have an associated iron deficiency anaemia (Chisholm *et al.* 1971). Pernicious anaemia, thyroid disease, ulcerative colitis and Sjogren's syndrome are other conditions which are associated with post-cricoid webs. Radiologically webs may be single or multiple and they are seen in the upper oesophagus, the most common site being at the level of the cricopharyngeal sphincter. Usually they are situated anteriorly but they can completely encircle the lumen. There is a high incidence of malignant lesions of the hypopharynx and oesophagus in patients with webs (Ekberg 1981).

Achalasia of the cardia

The aetiology of achalasia of the cardia is unknown. The condition is presumed to be due to the absence or degeneration of the ganglion cells in Meissner's and Auerbach's plexus (Barrett 1964). The cardinal changes that typify achalasia are disappearance of normal oesophageal peristalsis and its replacement by uncoordinated movements, failure of the cardia to relax, distortion and hypertrophy of the oesophagus above the cardia and an increased sensitivity of the oesophagus to cholinergic drugs (Adams *et al.* 1961). Patients with achalasia cannot swallow in the head-down position. The normal gas bubble of the fundus is generally absent.

The presenting symptoms are a choking feeling on attempting to swallow, difficulty in swallowing, regurgitation of food and saliva, vomiting, precordial pain and hunger (Barrett 1964). The early changes observed radiologically are absence of normal peristalsis in the oesophagus and its replacement by strong uncoordinated movements combined with poor emptying of the oesophagus when the patient is horizontal on the X-ray table. In an advanced case there is dilatation of the whole oesophagus with tapering of the distal 2–3 cm; a large amount of food and fluid may be present in the dilated oesophagus. Tumours such as carcinomas and leiomyomas occur more frequently than usual in the dilated oesophagus (Barrett 1964).

Infiltrating carcinoma of the oesophagus can simulate achalasia of the cardia and the radiological distinction between the two conditions can be very difficult (Lawson & Dodds 1976). All patients with suspected achalasia should undergo manometric studies and endoscopy with biopsy to confirm the diagnosis.

Chagas' disease (South American trypanosomiasis) causes similar changes in the oesophagus to achalasia.

Diffuse oesophageal spasm

There are three well-defined groups of patients who suffer oesophageal spasm (Gonzalez 1973). It may be a manifestation of gastro-oesophageal reflux and oesophagitis in some patients. In others it occurs due to the ageing process or various central nervous system diseases. The third group are patients in whom oesophageal spasm is the manifestation of a primary disease process. Substernal discomfort simulating cardiac pain may be experienced (Zaino & Beneventano 1977). On radiological examination the primary peristaltic wave is suddenly replaced by segmental uncoordinated contractions involving the lower third of the oesophagus. When spasm is due to a primary disease segmental contractions produce pseudodiverticula with a typical corkscrew appearance. There may also be evidence of thickening of the wall of the oesophagus in this group.

Muscular disorders

There are a number of uncommon conditions that cause muscular disorders of the oesophagus. Dystrophia myotonica may cause the oesophagus to dilate throughout its length similar to achalasia (Goldberg & Sheft 1972). Amyloid, deposited in the oesophageal musculature, may cause loss of peristalsis and megaoesophagus (Miller 1969). Scleroderma may diminish peristaltic activity, resulting eventually in complete absence of normal contractability (Zaino & Beneventano 1977). The lower oesophageal sphincter becomes incompetent and this leads to free gastric reflux, oesophagitis and stricture formation.

Perforation

Oesophageal perforation is a serious condition resulting from trauma, usually following instrumentation. Endoscopy is the most common cause of oesophageal perforation (Berry & Ochsner 1973). Rupture of the oesophagus occurs during endoscopy in slightly less than 0.1 per cent of patients (Love & Berkow 1978). Perforation can also result from attempts to dilate strictures or narrowed segments of oesophagus. Anastomotic leaks may develop following the surgical repair of oesophageal lesions. Oesophageal perforation can be caused by indwelling balloon catheters, meat or fish bones, post-emetic trauma (Boerhaave's syndrome), blunt trauma and penetrating trauma (Love & Berkow 1978).

Plain radiographs are the initial investigation in suspected oesophageal perforation. Evidence of subcutaneous emphysema and sometimes anterior displacement of the trachea due to mediastinal emphysema is seen when the cervical oesophagus is perforated (Love & Berkow 1978). Perforation of the mid oesophagus results in the early appearance of mediastinal emphysema. Similar changes may be present when the distal oesophagus is perforated; a left pleural effusion often associated with a left pneumothorax is a frequent finding. The V sign of Naclerio, a triangular lucency seen through the heart, may be seen in lower oesophageal perforation (Parkin 1973).

Water-soluble contrast medium is useful for establishing the diagnosis and locating the site of perforation. Barium is advocated for giving superior definition by Meyers & Ghahremani (1975). An accurate localization of the site of perforation can be obtained by passing a tube to the stomach and injecting contrast medium as the tube is withdrawn (Kerr 1962).

Other conditions

Moniliasis is an inflammatory condition resulting from infection with the fungus *Candida albicans* causing ulceration and pseudomembrane formation in the oesophagus. It occurs mostly in patients with debilitating disease, particularly if they are being treated with steroids, antibiotics or immunosuppressive agents. The classical symptoms are pain on swallowing, often associated with persistent retrosternal pain (Holt 1968). There is poor peristalsis and slow transit of barium through the oesophagus with limited distensibility and motility (Gonzalez 1971). The oesophageal mucosa is irregular and shaggy and if the contrast medium penetrates the pseudomembrane a double contour may be seen. Nodular irregular filling defects may be seen giving a cobblestone appearance (Goldberg & Dodds 1968). The ulcers and their margins are particularly well outlined on double-contrast barium examinations (Nolan 1980).

Acanthosis nigricans can involve the oesophagus; it is seen on double-contrast barium examination as fine nodular filling defects throughout the oesophagus (Itai *et al.* 1976). It is also possible to show leukoplakia of the oesophagus as small superficial protrusions with unsharp margins (Itai *et al.* 1977). Herpes oesophagitis may show changes that resemble moniliasis on double-contrast views of the oesophagus (Skucas *et al.* 1977).

References

Adams C.W.M., Brain R.H.F., Ellis F.G., Kauntze R. & Trounce J.R. (1961) Achalasia of the cardia. *Guy Hosp. Rep.*, **110**, 191

Banfield W.J. & Hurwitz A.L. (1974) Oesophageal stricture associated with nasogastric intubation. *Arch. Intern. Med.*, **134**, 1083

Barrett N.R. (1950) Chronic peptic ulcer of the oesophagus and 'oesophagitis'. *Br. J. Surg.*, **38**, 175

Barrett N.R. (1964) Achalasia of the cardia: Reflections upon a clinical study of over 100 cases. *Br. Med. J.*, **i**, 1135

Berry B.E. & Ochsner J.L. (1973) Perforation of the oesophagus—a 30 year review. *J. Thorac. Cardiovasc. Surg.*, **65**, 1

Chisholm M., Ardran G.M., Callender S.T. & Wright R. (1971) A follow-up study of patients with post-cricoid webs. *Q. J. Med.*, **40**, 409

Cho S.-R., Sanders M.M., Turner M.A., Liu C.-I. & Kipreos B.E. (1981) Oesophageal intramural pseudodiverticulosis. *Gastrointest. Radiol.*, **6**, 9

Cross F.S., Johnson G.F. & Gerein A.N. (1961) Oesophageal diverticula. Associated neuromuscular changes in the oesophagus. *Arch. Surg.*, **83**, 525

Dyer N.H., Cook P.L. & Kemp Harper R.A. (1969) Oesophageal stricture associated with Crohn's disease. *Gut*, **10**, 549

Ekberg O. (1981) Cervical oesophageal webs in patients with dysphagia. *Clin. Radiol.*, **32**, 633

Goldberg H.I. & Dodds J.W. (1968) Cobblestone oesophagus due to monilial infection. *Am. J. Roentgenol.*, **104**, 608

Goldberg H.I. & Sheft D.J. (1972) Oesophageal and colon changes in dystrophia myotonica. *Gastroenterology*, **63**, 134

Gonzalez G. (1971) Oesophageal moniliasis. *Am. J. Roentgenol.*, **113**, 233

Gonzalez G. (1973) Diffuse oesophageal spasm. *Am. J. Roentgenol.* **117**, 251

Goyal R.K., Bauer J.I. & Spiro H.H. (1971) The nature and location of lower oesophageal ring. *N. Engl. J. Med.*, **284**, 1175

Holt J.M. (1968) *Candida* infection of the oesophagus. *Gut*, **9**, 227

Itai Y., Kogure T., Okuyama Y. & Akiyama H. (1976) Radiological manifestations of oesophageal involvement in acanthosis nigricans. *Br. J. Radiol.*, **49**, 592

Itai Y., Kogure T., Okuyama Y. & Akiyama H. (1977) Diffuse finely nodular lesions of the oesophagus. *Am. J. Roentgenol.*, **128**, 563

Kerr I.H. (1962) A method of demonstrating the site of a perforation of the oesophagus. *Br. J. Radiol.*, **35**, 255

Kressel H.Y., Glick S.N., Laufer I. & Banner M. (1981) Radiologic features of oesophagitis. *Gastrointest. Radiol.*, **6**, 103

Lawson T.L. & Dodds W.J. (1976) Infiltrating carcinoma simulating achalasia. *Gastrointest. Radiol.*, **1**, 245

Love L. & Berkow A.E. (1978) Trauma to the oesophagus. *Gastrointest. Radiol.*, **2**, 305

Lunderquist A. & Vang J. (1974) Transhepatic catheterization and obliteration of the coronary vein in patients with portal hypertension and oesophageal varices. *N. Engl. J. Med.*, **291**, 646

Meyers M.A. & Ghahremani G.G. (1975) Complications of fibreoptic endoscopy. *Radiology*, **115**, 293

Miller R.H. (1969) Amyloid disease—an unusual case of megaloesophagus. *S. Afr. Med. J.*, **43**, 1202

Morson B.C. & Dawson I.M.P. (1979) *Gastrointestinal Pathology*. Oxford: Blackwell Scientific Publications

Nolan D.J. (1980) *The Double-Contrast Barium Meal— A Radiological Atlas*. Aylesbury: HM + M

Parkin G.J.S. (1973) The radiology of perforated oesophagus. *Clin. Radiol.*, **24**, 324

Rogers L.F. & Goldstein H.M. (1977) Roentgen manifestations of radiation injury to the gastrointestinal tract. *Gastrointest. Radiol.*, **2**, 281

Schneider R. (1976) Tuberculous oesophagitis. *Gastrointest. Radiol.*, **1**, 143

Sherlock S. (1981) *Diseases of the Liver and Biliary System*. Oxford: Blackwell Scientific Publications

Shirazi K.K., Daffner R.H. & Gaede J.T. (1977) Ulcer occurring in Zenker's diverticulum. *Gastrointest. Radiol.*, **2**, 117

Skucas J., Schrank W.W., Meyers P.C. & Lee C.S. (1977) Herpes oesophagitis. A case studied by air-contrast oesophagography. *Am. J. Roentgenol.*, **128**, 497

Spiro H.M. (1977) *Clinical Gastroenterology*. New York: Macmillan

Wynder E.L. & Bross I.J. (1961) A study of aetiological factors in cancer of the oesophagus. *Cancer*, **14**, 389

Zaino C. & Beneventano T.C. (1977) *Radiologic Examination of the Orohypopharynx and Oesophagus*. New York: Springer-Verlag

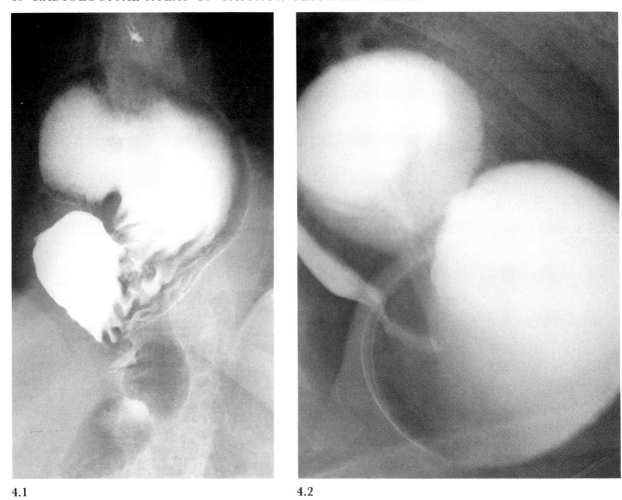

4.1

4.2

4.1 **Hiatal hernia** A large sliding type hiatal hernia is shown. All the stomach except the distal antrum has herniated into the thorax

4.2 **Hiatal hernia** There is a large rolling type hiatal hernia causing volvulus of the stomach. As a result barium did not pass into the duodenum for at least an hour. This 67-year-old woman presented with vomiting. A transthoracic repair of the hiatal hernia was performed

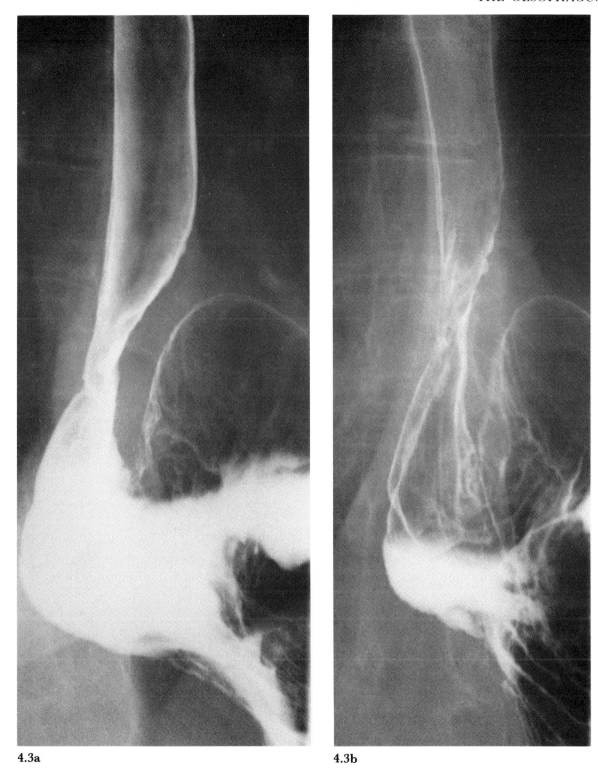

4.3a

4.3b

4.3 **Hiatal hernia and peptic oesophagitis** a,b A moderate-sized hiatal hernia and narrowing and ulceration of the lower oesophagus are seen

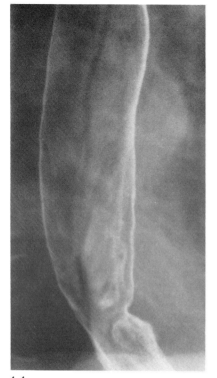

4.4

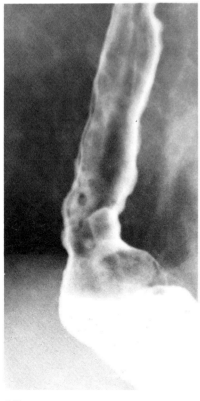

4.5

4.6

4.4 **Peptic oesophagitis** A short segment of the lower oesophagus is narrowed with irregularity and some nodularity of the walls, and there are a number of thickened mucosal folds

4.5 **Hiatal hernia and peptic oesophagitis** A small hiatal hernia is seen; gastro-oesophageal reflux occurred during the examination. There is also irregularity, ulceration, nodularity and a small number of thickened folds

4.6 Hiatal hernia and junctional ulcer An ulcer crater (arrow) is seen at the oesophagogastric junction in a patient with a sliding type hiatal hernia who was admitted with upper gastrointestinal bleeding. The ulcer was also seen at endoscopy and confirmed at operation

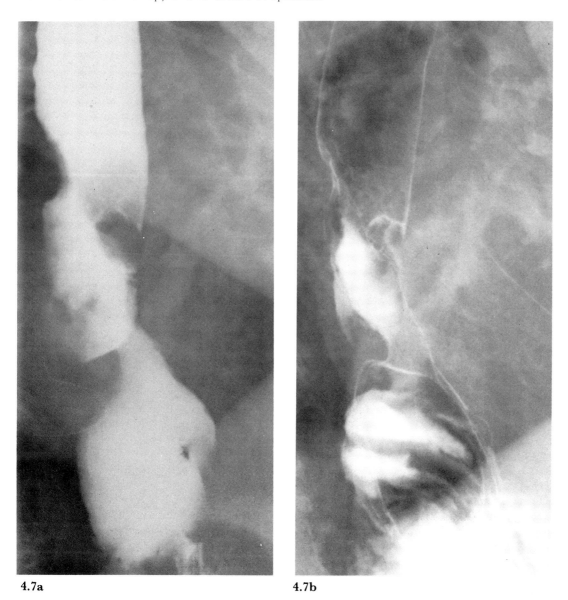

4.7a

4.7b

4.7 Hiatal hernia and junctional ulcer a,b A large oval ulcer, with an oedematous margin, is shown just above a hiatal hernia. The patient, an 88-year-old woman, was admitted with haematemesis. Biopsies obtained at endoscopy showed no evidence of malignancy. The ulcer healed following medical treatment and the patient remained well 18 months later

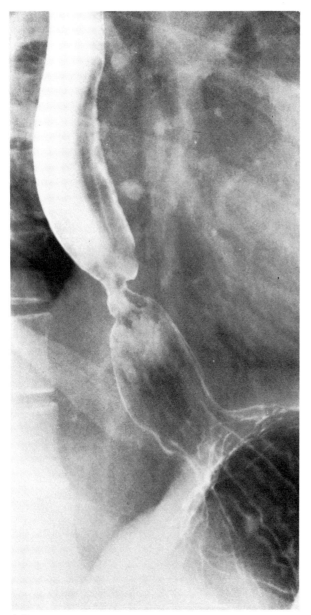

4.8

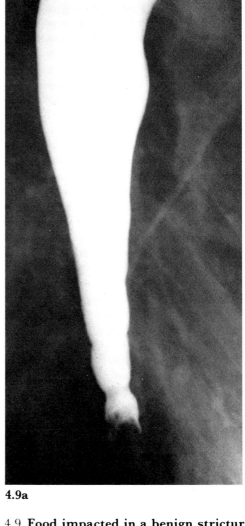

4.9a

4.8 Hiatal hernia and peptic stricture There is a short segment of irregular narrowing with smooth margins and minimal ulceration in the lower oesophagus. A small hiatal hernia is also seen. The diagnosis of a benign stricture was confirmed on biopsies obtained at endoscopy

4.9 Food impacted in a benign stricture a A filling defect is causing complete obstruction in a narrowed segment of distal oesophagus. b A long slightly irregular, benign peptic stricture of the lower oesophagus is shown on a view taken at a repeat examination, after removal of the impacted food bolus

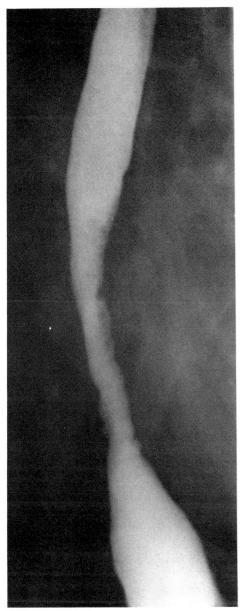

4.9b

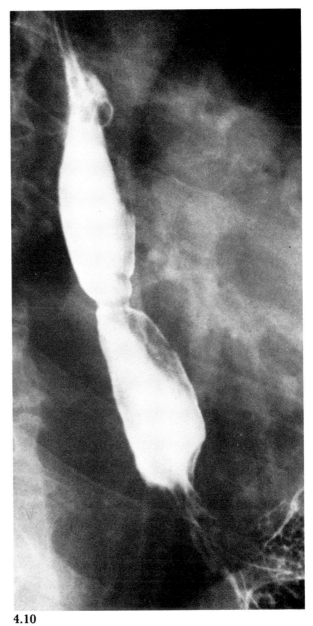

4.10

4.10 **Benign peptic stricture** There is a very short
segment of narrowing, about 3 mm long, in the
distal oesophagus of a 59-year-old man with a
known history of gastro-oesophageal reflux who was
examined because of chest pain. The oesophageal
narrowing was not causing any symptoms. He
proved to have coronary artery disease on
angiography

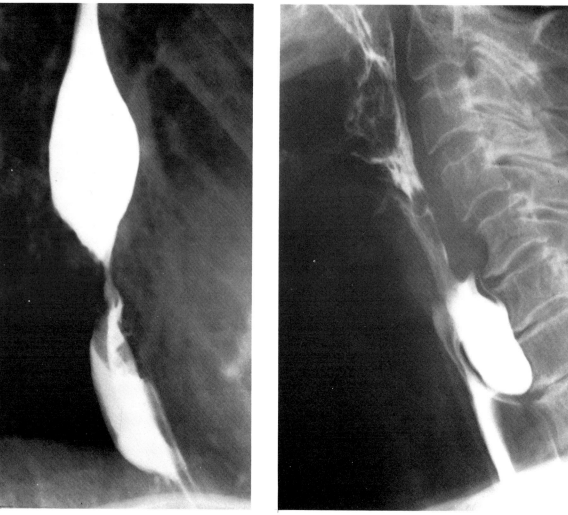

4.11a

4.11b

4.11 **Benign peptic stricture and Zenker's diverticulum** a A segment of distal oesophagus is grossly narrowed and irregular. b This view of the upper oesophagus shows a moderate-sized Zenker's diverticulum. The patient, an elderly female, presented with dysphagia. Endoscopy which was subsequently attempted with caution in order to obtain biopsies from the narrowed segment proved impossible because of the diverticulum. When endoscopy was repeated after the Zenker's diverticulum had been resected there was evidence of a benign stricture in the distal oesophagus

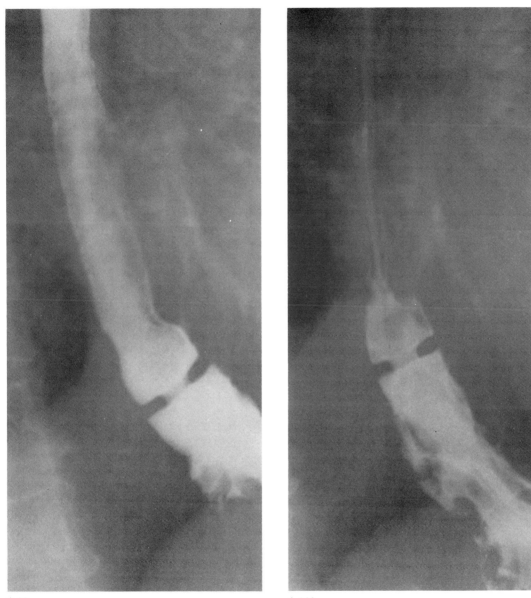

4.12a

4.12b

4.12 **Schatzki ring** a,b A constant ring-like
constriction is seen at the distal end of the
oesophagus. There is also a small hiatal hernia.
(Courtesy of Mr. A. Gunning)

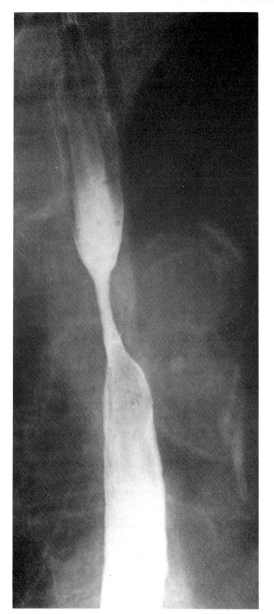

4.13

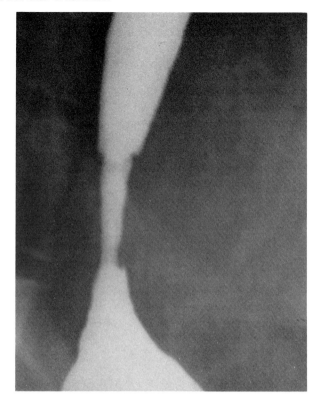

4.14a

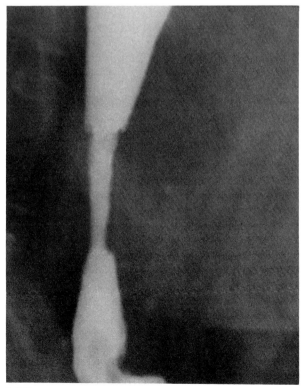

4.14b

4.13 **Benign stricture** A narrowed segment with smooth margins, about 3 cm in length, is seen at the level of the aortic arch. The narrowing was constant on all views. The 84-year-old woman presented with a six- month history of increasing dysphagia. A mid oesophageal stricture with mild oesophagitis was confirmed at endoscopy. The oesophagus distal to the stricture was of normal calibre and was lined by normal squamous epithelium

4.14 **Peptic stricture resulting from prolonged nasogastric intubation** a,b A short tight stricture, about 3 cm long, is shown by the barium column in the lower oesophagus. A small hiatal hernia with free gastro-oesophageal reflux was also seen. The 55-year-old woman who was admitted to hospital three weeks earlier had been fed for nine days via a nasogastric tube because of persistent vomiting due to hepatic failure. The stricture was dilated endoscopically. Barium studies and endoscopy performed during a previous admission six months before showed a hiatal hernia and oesophagitis but no evidence of stricture formation

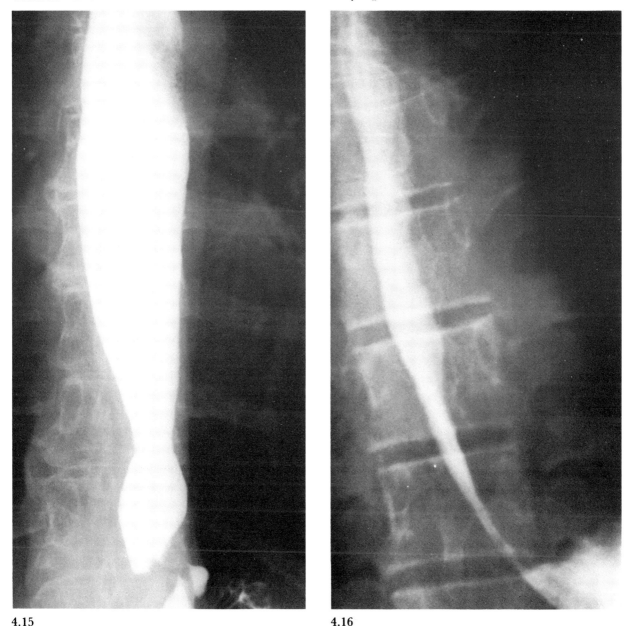

4.15

4.16

4.15 **Oesophageal stricture in a patient with scleroderma** A short segment of narrowing, constant on all views, is shown in the lower oesophagus of a 51-year-old woman with scleroderma. A small hiatal hernia can also be seen. The oesophagus did not empty while the patient was horizontal. Hiatal hernia with gastro-oesophageal reflux resulting in stricture formation is a well recognized complication of scleroderma. (Courtesy of Dr. Myles McNulty)

4.16 **Corrosive stricture** There is a long tapered, slightly irregular narrowing of the mid and lower oesophagus. This young man swallowed hydrochloric acid in a suicide attempt. (Courtesy of Dr. Stuart Field)

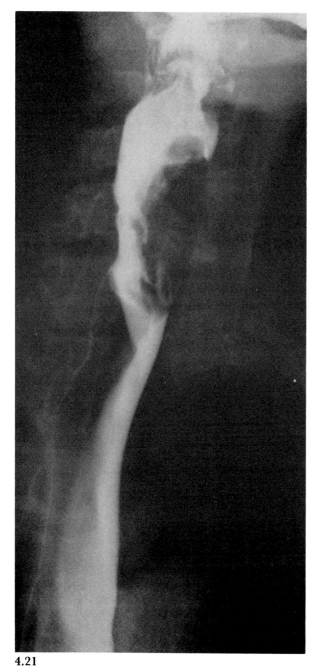

4.21

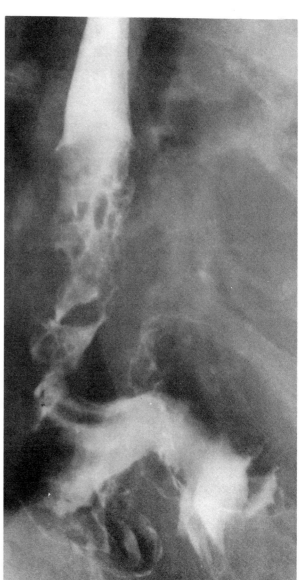

4.22

4.21 **Carcinoma** There is a large irregular filling defect occupying the left side of the upper oesophagus in a patient who presented with dysphagia. Endoscopy and examination of biopsy specimens confirmed the diagnosis

4.22 **Carcinoma** There is an irregular polypoid mass involving a long segment of the lower oesophagus. A hiatal hernia is also seen in this 79-year-old man who presented with abdominal pain and anorexia. The lesion proved to be a moderately well-differentiated adenocarcinoma

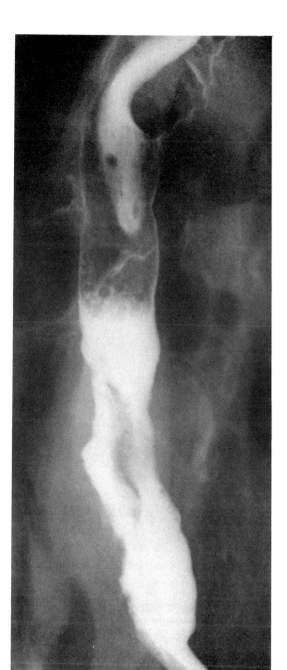

4.23

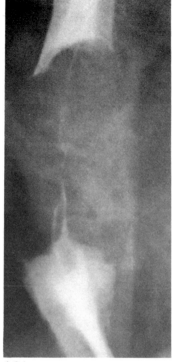

4.24

4.24 Infiltrating carcinoma There is marked narrowing of a segment of lower oesophagus in an elderly man who presented with dysphagia. Shouldering of the upper margin is seen

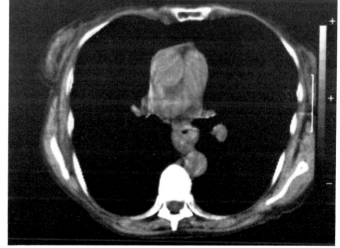

4.25

4.23 Carcinoma There is a large ulcerating lesion in the lower oesophagus with narrowing of the lumen and an associated soft tissue mass. The 80-year-old man was admitted to hospital in a weak state and gave a history of dysphagia and weight loss. He died before further investigations could be performed

4.25 Carcinoma shown on CT Marked thickening and an irregular outline of the wall of the oesophagus is shown on a *computed tomography scan* in a patient with carcinoma of the oesophagus. (Courtesy of Department of Diagnostic Imaging, Royal Marsden Hospital)

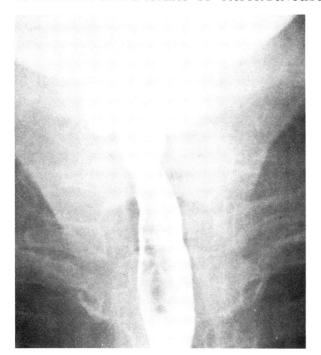

4.41a

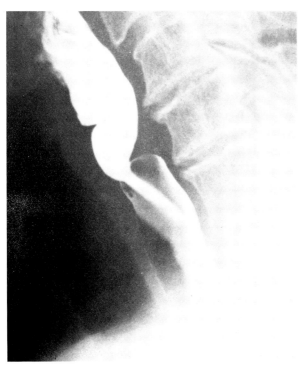

4.41b

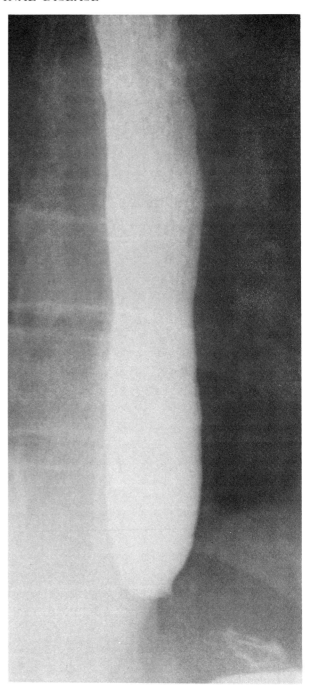

4.42

4.41 **Oesophageal webs** a,b Two post-cricoid webs are shown, the upper one is situated anteriorly and the lower one encircles the lumen. A narrow jet of barium is seen passing downwards from the lower web on the lateral view

4.42 **Achalasia of the cardia** A tapered narrowing of the lower oesophagus is seen. There was a delay in oesophageal emptying and uncoordinated movements were noticed on fluoroscopy. The patient, a 29-year-old female, presented with dysphagia. The diagnosis was subsequently confirmed

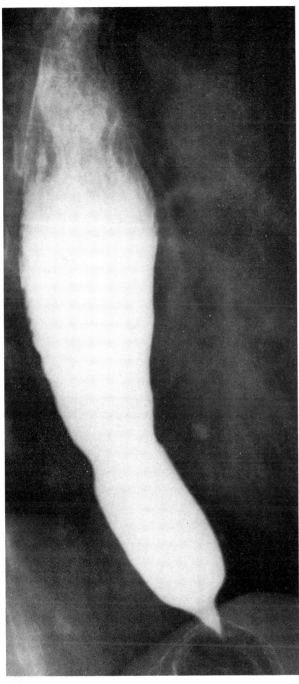

4.43a

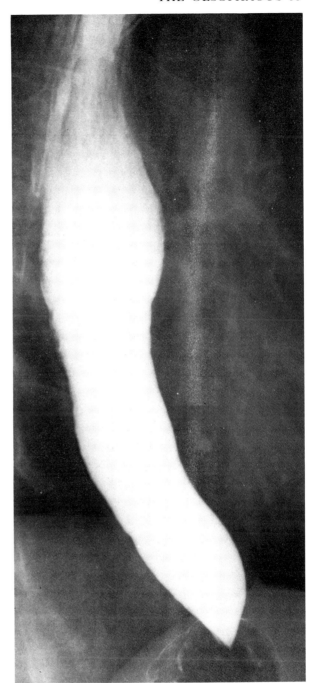

4.43b

4.43 Achalasia of the cardia a,b There is tapered narrowing of the distal end of the oesophagus. Slight dilatation of the oesophagus can also be seen. There was considerable delay in emptying of the oesophagus and abnormal peristaltic activity was seen on fluoroscopy. This 45-year-old woman presented with dyspepsia. On further questioning she gave a history of increasing dysphagia for solids and liquids, regurgitation of food and slight weight loss. Achalasia of the cardia was confirmed at endoscopy

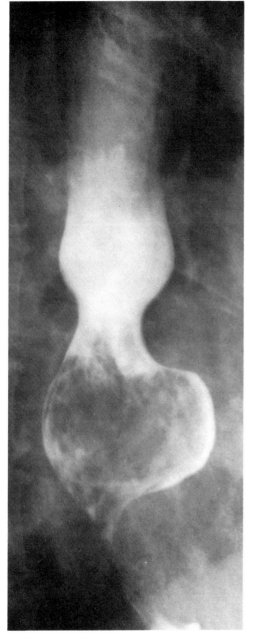

4.44a

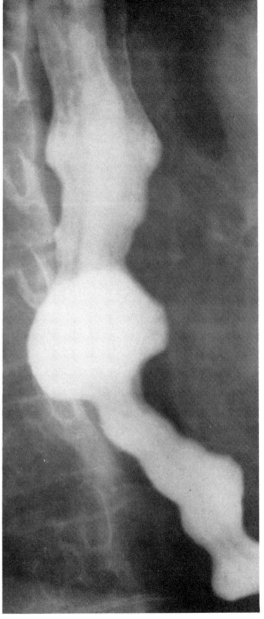

4.44b

4.44 **Oesophageal spasm** a A large bolus of food is impacted in the lower oesophagus. b Diffuse oesophageal spasm (tertiary contractions) is seen throughout the lower half of the oesophagus at the repeat examination after removal of the food bolus

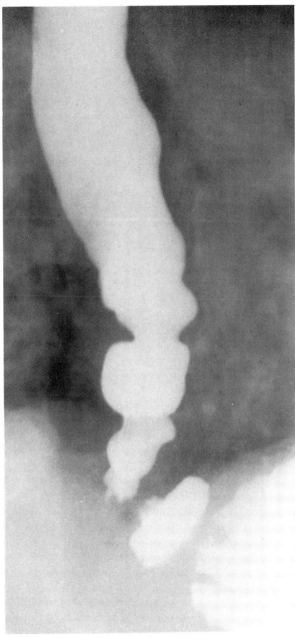

4.45

4.45 **'Corkscrew' oesophagus** Diffuse
oesophageal spasm (tertiary contractions)
is seen in the lower oesophagus giving the
typical 'corkscrew' appearance

4.46 **Amyloid disease** A view showing
megaoesophagus in a 67-year-old man
with established amyloid disease for two
years. Absence of peristalsis was noted on
fluoroscopy

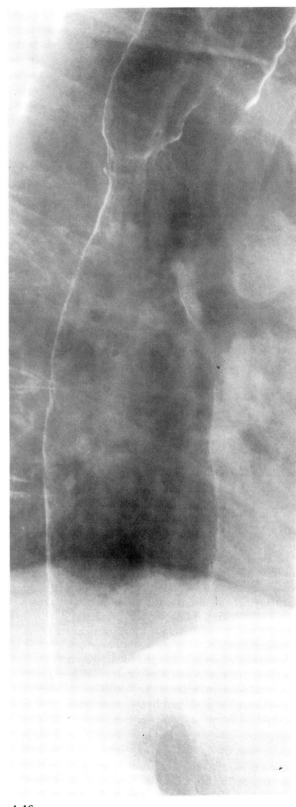

4.46

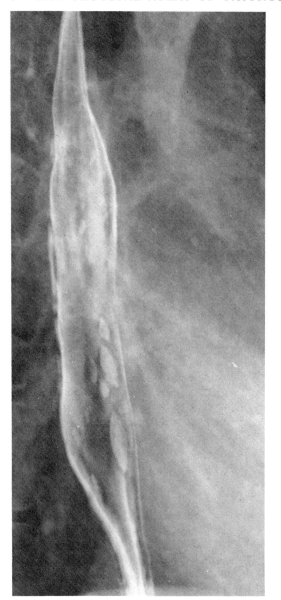
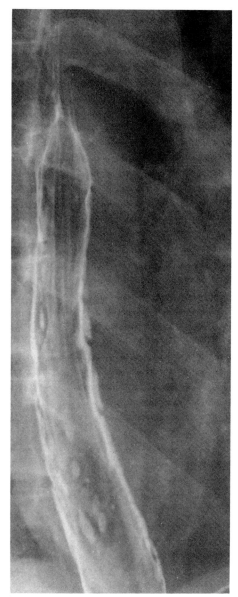

4.50a   **4.50b**

4.50 **Moniliasis** a,b Mucosal ulcers in the distal half of the oesophagus are seen *en face* and in profile. A radiolucent border, presumably due to oedema, surrounds each ulcer. The 24-year-old man developed dysphagia following an emergency colectomy for acute Crohn's colitis. White plaques of *Candida albicans* together with punched out ulcers and oesophagitis were seen at endoscopy. There was an immediate symptomatic improvement on treatment with nystatin and a follow-up examination showed that the ulcers had healed

Peptic ulceration

A peptic ulcer is a circumscribed lesion involving loss of the full thickness of the mucosa and a variable amount of underlying tissue (Morson & Dawson 1979). The stomach and duodenum are the predominant sites of benign peptic ulceration. A recent study showed that gastric ulceration occurred in a male/female ratio of 1.9:1 (Montgomery 1977). According to that report the disease is rare under the age of 20 years, with the maximum number of patients presenting in the sixth and seventh decades of life. Gastric ulcers were multiple in 6 per cent and there were associated duodenal ulcers in 15 per cent of cases.

Gastric ulcers may be acute or chronic. Some scarring will occur initially when an acute ulcer heals, but after a few weeks the site of the original ulcer is difficult or impossible to find (Truelove & Reynell 1972). A chronic peptic ulcer possesses much fibrous tissue and cellular infiltration in its floor and margins. It is slower to heal than an acute ulcer and results in considerable scarring. Healing of a long-established chronic ulcer is a difficult process as the newly formed mucosa is likely to break down into a fresh ulcer.

Aspirin and indomethacin are drugs commonly associated with gastric ulceration. Indomethacin, at least in high doses, is ulcerogenic (Wigley & Fowles 1976). On the evidence available, corticosteroids in low doses do not seem to increase the incidence of ulcers. The risk is probably greater if they are combined with other analgesics. Large doses of corticosteroids in acute illness, where other factors are operating, may cause gastric ulceration. Acute ulcers are common in old age. They are often associated with chronic lung disease and malignancy, in particular bronchial carcinoma. There is a low incidence in patients with fatal coronary artery disease (Montgomery 1977). Complications of gastric ulceration include haemorrhage, perforation, and penetration into adjacent organs such as the pancreas, liver and transverse colon. Stricture formation or sustained spasm may give the stomach an hourglass configuration (Montgomery 1977).

Gastric ulcers vary considerably in size. The most frequent site of ulceration is along the lesser curve and on the posterior wall (Diagram 5.1). The distribution of gastric ulcers found at endoscopy is similar, with as many occurring in the upper half of the stomach as in the lower half (Stevenson 1977). Greater-curve gastric ulcers are uncommon and are nearly always benign (Lumsden 1973; Kottler & Tuft 1981). They occur in the elderly, many of whom have concomitant disease and are taking multiple oral medication and analgesics (Kottler & Tuft 1981). These ulcers are prone to occasional perforation with the formation of gastrocolic fistula. The 26 greater-curve ulcers reported by Kottler & Tuft were all in the distal third of the greater curve. They were described as 'sump' ulcers because they were sited in the part of the stomach that was lowest when the patient was upright. Converging folds may be shown when healing has occurred. The authors suggest that tablets

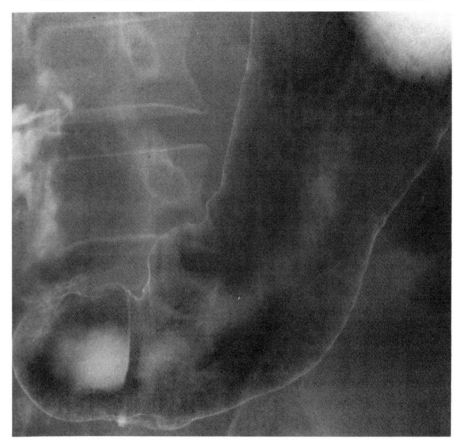

5.14a

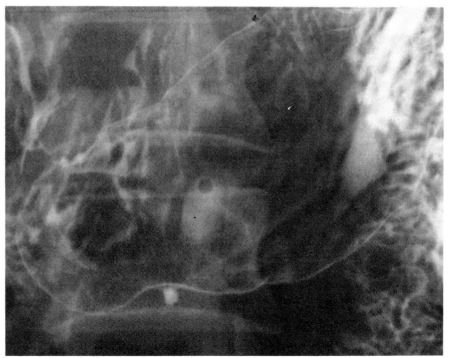

5.14b

5.14 **Sump ulcer** a,b
Double-contrast views show a
small ulcer crater situated
on the greater-curve aspect
of the antrum. c On a
compression single-contrast view
there is oedema around the
margins of the crater. The
patient developed
abdominal pain after taking
salicylate analgesics for
headache. Following a
course of medical treatment
endoscopy was performed
and the ulcer was found to
have healed completely

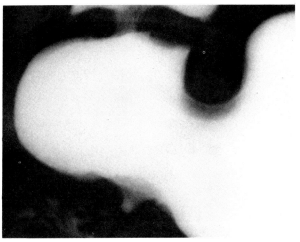

5.14c

5.15 **Bleeding peptic ulcer** A giant lesser-curve gastric ulcer, 8 cm × 6 cm, contains air and blood mixed with barium. The patient, an 81-year-old woman, collapsed and died ten hours later following a further episode of bleeding. Autopsy confirmed the presence of a giant benign ulcer

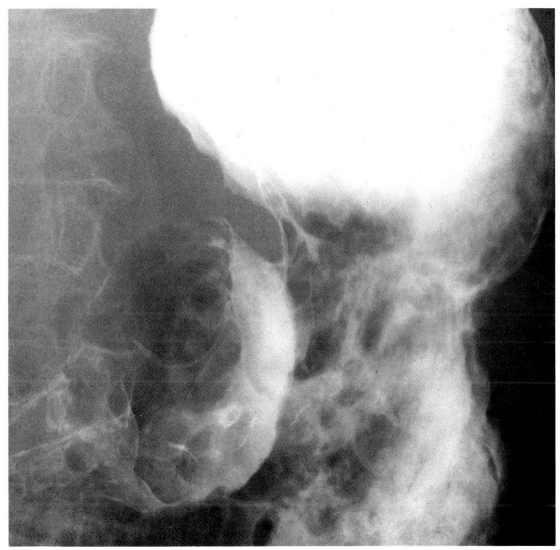

5.15

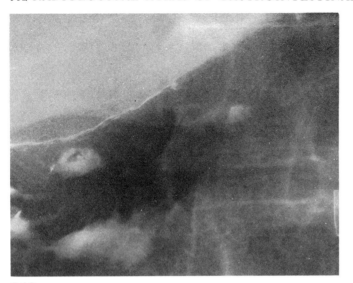

5.16

5.16 Peptic ulcer and 'Berg's nodule' Two gastric ulcers are shown in a patient who was admitted with melaena. An irregular translucent filling defect in the larger ulcer is due to the presence of blood clot—'Berg's nodule'. The patient responded to conservative treatment

5.17 Penetrating gastric ulcer and duodenal ulcer a A *double-contrast view* of the body of the stomach shows a lesser-curve gastric ulcer, 5 cm in diameter. b The nodular pattern in the base of the ulcer crater is an appearance often seen in gastric ulcers that penetrate the pancreas. c There is an ulcer, 1.5 cm in diameter, in the duodenal cap which is shown best on a *single-contrast view*

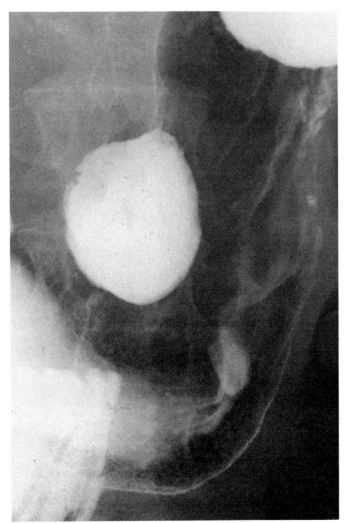

5.17a

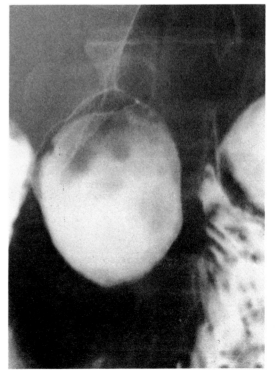

5.17b

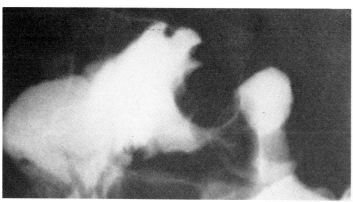

5.17c

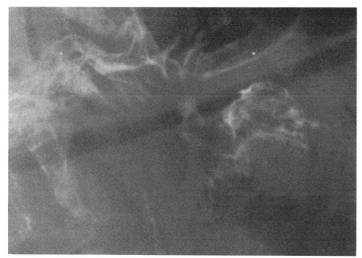

5.18

5.18 Penetrating peptic ulcer with gastrojejunal fistula A greater-curve sump ulcer with radiating mucosal folds is shown. Some barium has passed from the ulcer crater into a loop of jejunum. The 83-year-old woman was taking analgesics for arthritis and presented with a history of several months discomfort followed by a few weeks of diarrhoea. There was good symptomatic response to medical treatment and endoscopy three months later showed a healed ulcer scar with an hourglass deformity of the stomach

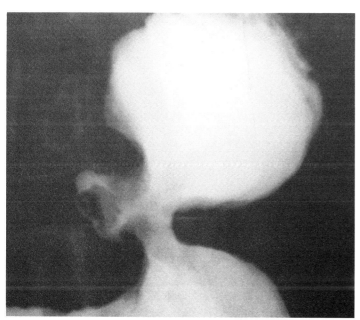

5.19

5.19 Peptic ulcer with hourglass deformity Marked contraction gives the stomach an hourglass deformity adjacent to a moderate-sized lesser curve gastric ulcer. A duodenal ulcer causing gastric outlet obstruction was also found. The patient, a 51-year-old woman with a long history of gastric ulceration, presented with recurrent dyspepsia. The gastric ulcer was found to be benign at operation

5.20 **Solitary erosion** There is a single erosion on a mucosal fold near the incisura angularis. The opaque area near the greater curve probably represents calcification in a mesenteric lymph gland

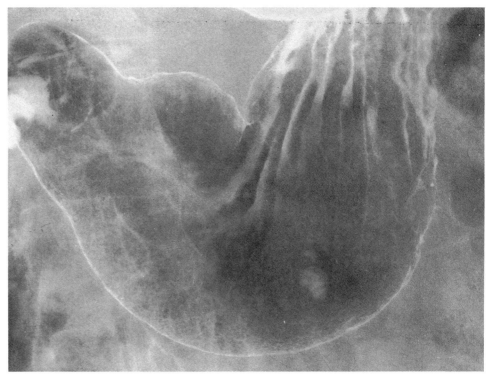

5.20

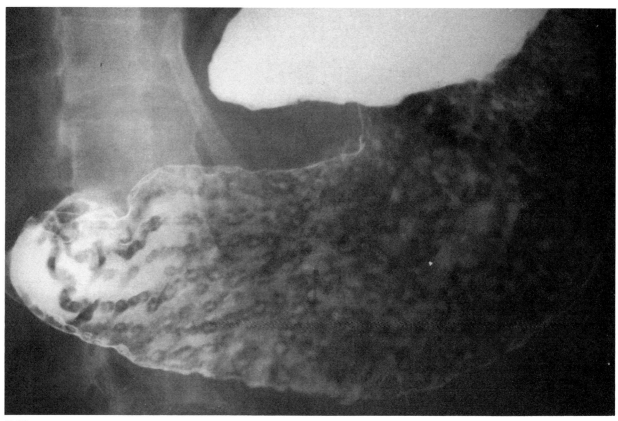

5.21a

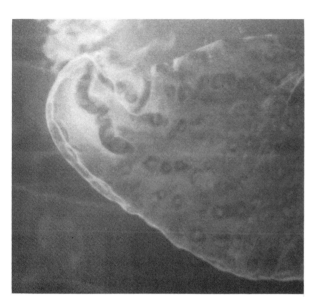

5.21b

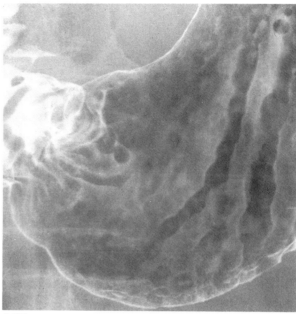

5.22a

5.21 **Erosive gastritis** a,b A large number of small and large erosions, with surrounding translucent zones due to oedema, are seen throughout the body and antrum of the stomach of a 32-year-old woman who presented with dyspepsia. The erosions were also seen at endoscopy. Examination of gastric biopsies and a normal small intestine ruled out the possibility of Crohn's disease. (Courtesy of Dr. I.S. Liyanage)

5.22 **Erosive gastritis** a Multiple small erosions with surrounding zones of oedema are present in the body and antrum of the stomach. At endoscopy round oedematous areas, 'like polyps with tiny ulcers in the centre', were seen. b Six months later there is a reduction in the number of erosions

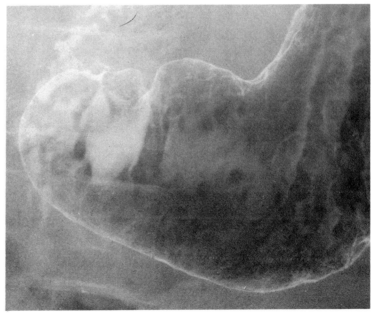

5.22b

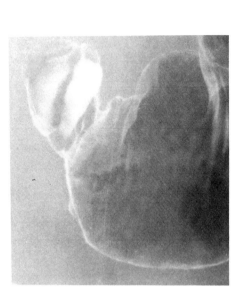

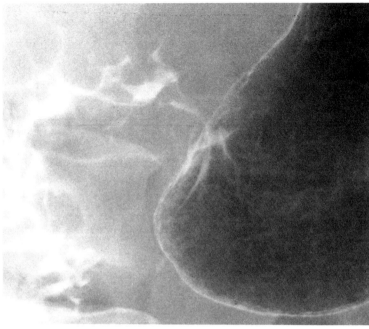

5.23

5.24

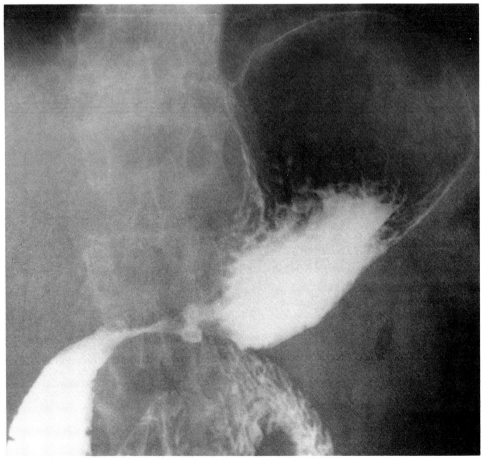

5.25a

5.23 **Antral gastritis** There is slight deformity of the prepyloric gastric antrum with a number of thickened mucosal folds. A small number of erosions are seen on one of the thickened folds. Similar appearances at endoscopy confirmed the diagnosis of antral gastritis

5.24 **Antral gastritis and pyloric stenosis** There is distortion and narrowing of the prepyloric gastric antrum, pylorus and duodenal cap and there was delay in the passage of barium into the duodenum. The patient, a 75-year-old man with a 50-year history of indigestion, presented with abdominal pain and vomiting. The prepyloric mucosa was irregular and the pylorus was narrowed at endoscopy. Histological examination of biopsies obtained showed evidence of chronic gastritis and intestinal metaplasia

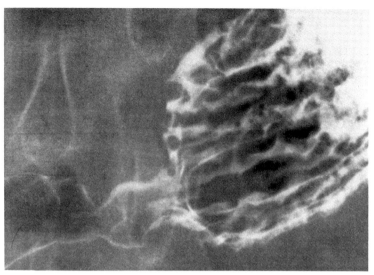

5.25b

5.25 **Anastomotic ulcer** a An ulcer crater, with oedema of the margins and associated deformity, is seen at a Billroth I anastomosis site. b Barium has emptied out of the ulcer which is situated anteriorly, leaving the ulcer crater outlined like a ring shadow. There was delay in the passage of barium into the duodenum. The 66-year-old man presented with abdominal pain and vomiting; his symptoms improved on medical treatment

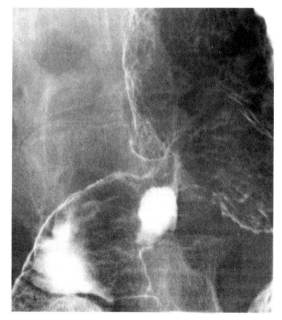

5.26

5.26 **Anastomotic ulcer** A moderate-sized ulcer crater is shown at the anastomosis site in a patient with a Billroth I partial gastrectomy who was admitted with melaena. A single-contrast barium examination and endoscopy failed to detect the ulcer but when endoscopy was repeated following this examination it was seen. The ulcer healed following a truncal vagotomy

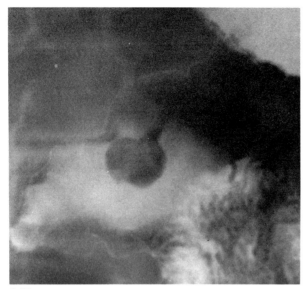

5.31

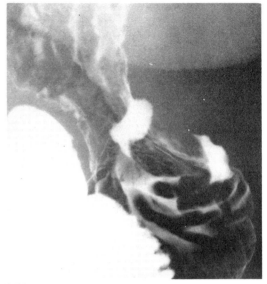

5.32

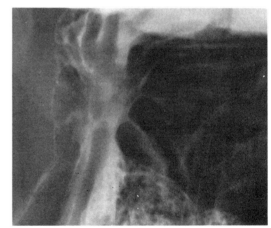

5.33a

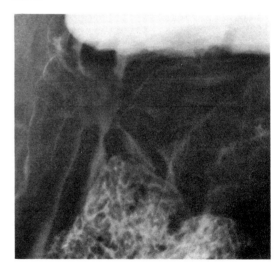

5.33b

5.31 **Pedunculated polyp** A large antral polyp on a short pedicle is outlined with a thin layer of barium. Endoscopy was not carried out because the patient, a 79-year-old man, was in severe congestive heart failure

5.32 **Ulcerating carcinoma** There is a moderate-sized ulcer crater in the body of the stomach near the greater curve in this 64-year-old woman who presented with epigastric pain. A poorly differentiated adenocarcinoma was diagnosed on biopsies obtained at endoscopy; an extensive carcinoma with metastases was found at operation

5.33 **Ulcerating carcinoma** a,b A shallow irregular ill-defined ulcer crater with an uneven floor is shown on the posterior wall of the upper body of the stomach. Some of the converging folds are distorted and fuse while others are widened and clubbed as they reach the edge of the ulcer. Histological examination of the resected specimen showed a poorly differentiated adenocarcinoma, mainly within the mucosa but in some areas spreading into the submucosa and through to the serosa. (Courtesy of Dr. J.C. MacLarnon)

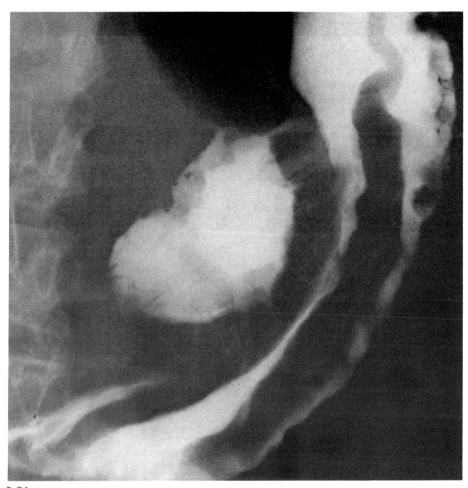

5.34a

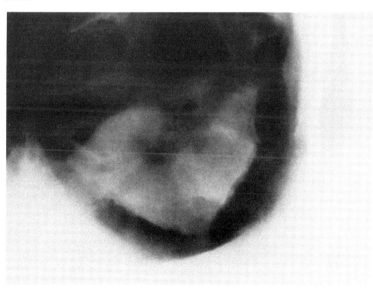

5.34b

5.34 **Ulcerating carcinoma** a There is a large lesser-curve gastric ulcer on a *single-contrast mucosal view* of the stomach. b *A compression view* shows the ulcer crater with the characteristic 'meniscus' sign. The 74-year-old man presented with severe sharp central abdominal pain, loss of energy and weight loss. A large poorly differentiated adenocarcinoma invading the serosa and with lymph node metastases was found at operation; a palliative gastrectomy was performed

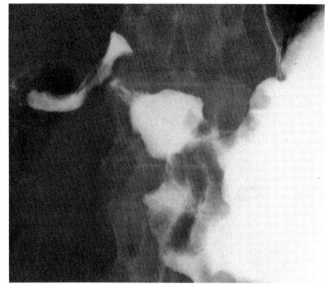

5.35

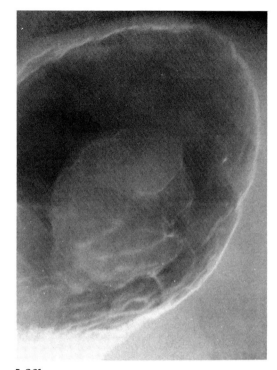

5.36b

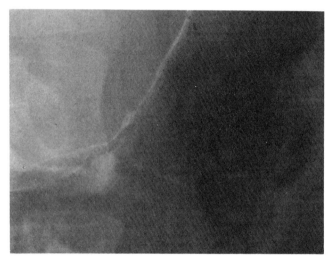

5.36a

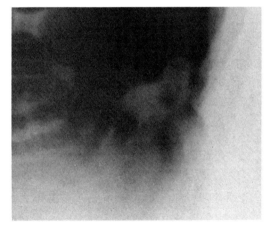

5.37a

5.35 Ulcerating antral carcinoma The gastric antrum is markedly narrowed and deformed and contains a moderate-sized ulcer crater that was shown best on this *single-contrast view*. The 65-year-old female presented with abdominal pain and had an abdominal mass on clinical examination. Biopsies obtained at endoscopy showed evidence of malignancy; an extensive adenocarcinoma was found at operation

5.36 Ulcerating carcinoma a This *double-contrast view* shows a poorly defined ulcer crater at the incisura angularis. b A *compression view* shows the ulcer with a meniscus shape, a slightly irregular outline and a nodular pattern around the margin. The ulcer was reported as likely to be malignant but direct inspection at operation suggested that it was benign. However, histological examination showed an ulcerating adenocarcinoma which was mainly intramucosal but showed some extension right out to the serosa

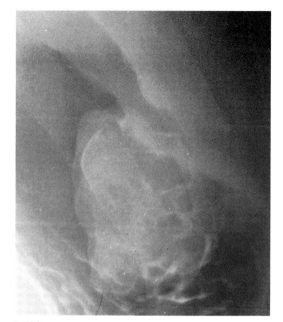

5.37b

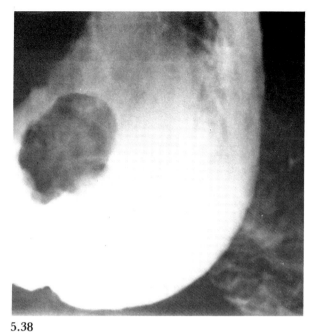

5.38

5.37 **Polypoid carcinoma** a,b A large irregular polypoid filling defect is seen attached to the posterior wall of the fundus of the stomach. The 67-year-old man, with a three-year history of angina, presented with melaena. Local excision of the carcinoma was performed and the limits of the excision showed normal mucosa with no evidence of infiltration. The patient remains well five years later

5.38 **Polypoid carcinoma** An irregular polypoid filling defect is shown at the junction of the body and antrum of the stomach on this *single-contrast view*. The 64-year-old man, with a 30-year-old history of pernicious anaemia, presented with dyspepsia. A polypoid adenocarcinoma was found at operation

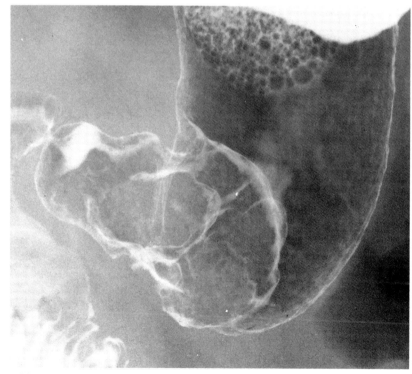

5.39

5.39 **Polypoid carcinoma** An irregular polypoid filling defect is shown involving the gastric antrum and distal part of the body of the stomach (Nolan 1978)

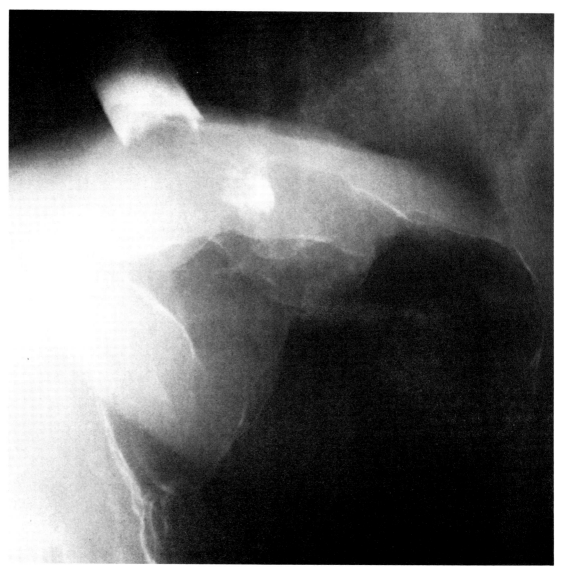

5.40

5.40 **Polypoid carcinoma** There is an extensive polypoid filling defect in the fundus of the stomach invading and obstructing the lower end of the oesophagus. A Celeston tube was inserted endoscopically as a palliative procedure in this 72-year-old man who presented with dysphagia

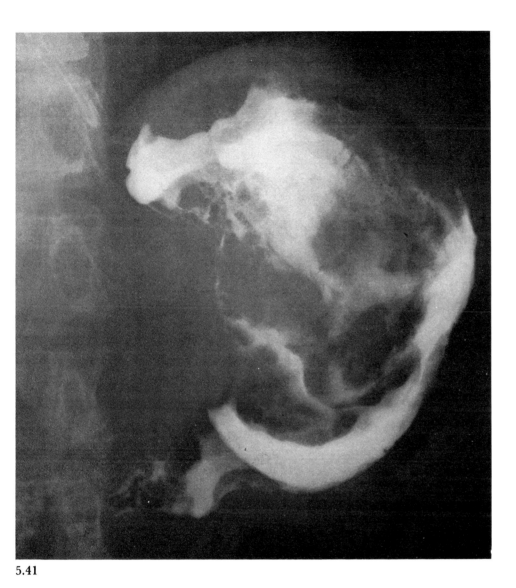

5.41

5.41 **Polypoid carcinoma** An extensive fungating carcinoma is seen
involving nearly all of the fundus and body of the stomach. This 84-year-old
man was admitted with epigastric discomfort, weight loss and anaemia

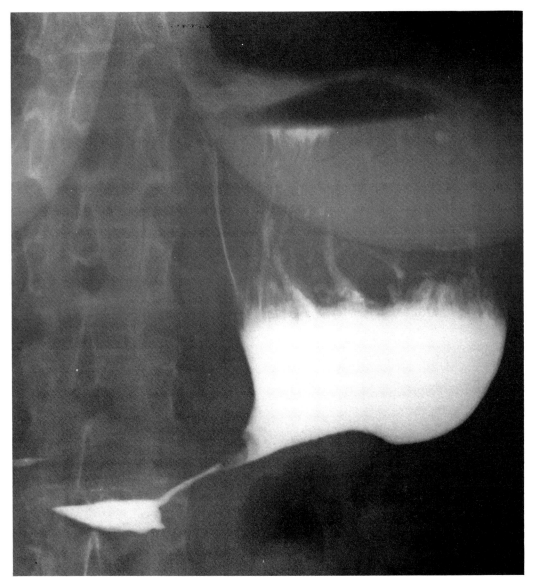

5.42

5.42 **Infiltrating carcinoma** A tight smooth stricture of the antrum and distal part of the stomach is outlined with barium. The 67-year-old woman with a 35-year history of pernicious anaemia was investigated because of abdominal pain, vomiting and weight loss. An extensive infiltrating carcinoma of the stomach, spreading to the lymph glands, was found at operation

5.43 **Linitis plastica** a,b *Single and double-contrast views* show loss of the normal mucosal pattern and contraction of the fundus, body and proximal antrum of the stomach. The 67-year-old woman presented with diffuse epigastric pain and weight loss. A widely infiltrating carcinoma was found at operation

5.44 **Linitis plastica** A *double-contrast view* shows that most of the stomach is contracted and has failed to distend. The mucosal pattern of the body of the stomach is irregular and distorted. The 58-year-old man presented with a three-month history of fullness in the stomach and weight loss of 14 lbs. The diagnosis was confirmed at operation and the stomach was resected. Pathological examination showed the typical appearance of linitis plastica ('leather bottle' stomach)

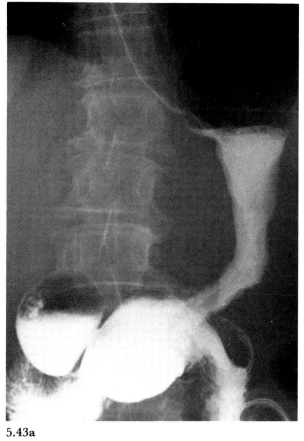

5.43a

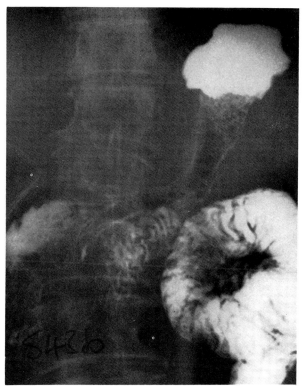

5.43b

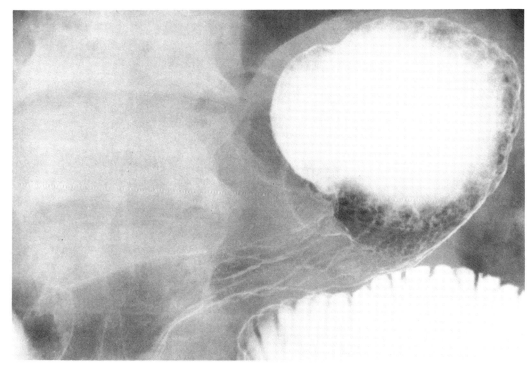

5.44

5.45 **Carcinoma following previous gastric surgery** There is an irregular infiltrating lesion causing narrowing and distortion at the anastomosis site in a 69-year-old man who 30 years earlier had a Polya-type partial gastrectomy. He presented with a four-month history of abdominal pain, weight loss and the recent onset of vomiting

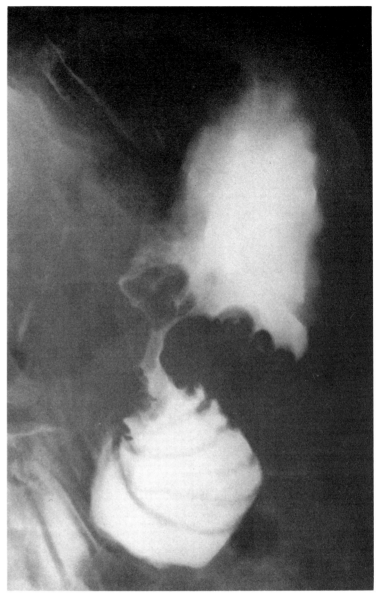

5.45

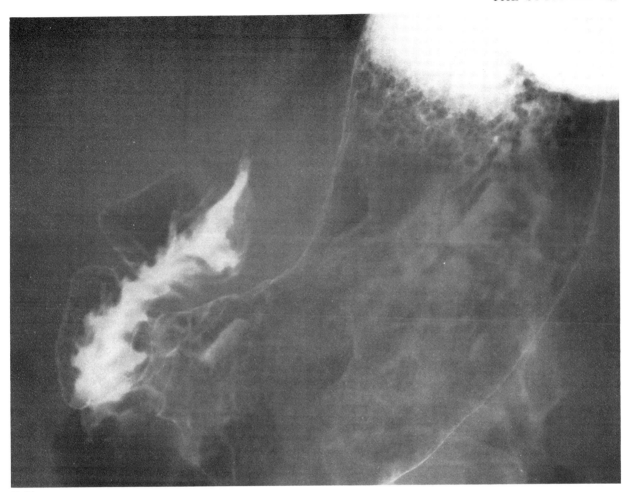

5.46a

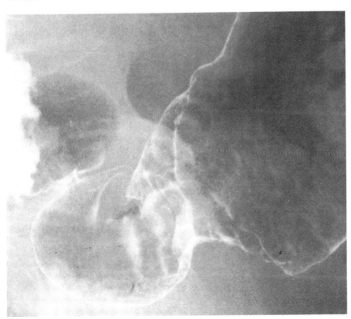

5.46b

5.46 **Early gastric cancer—type IIb** a,b Most of the gastric antrum is irregular in outline, slightly narrowed and the mucosal pattern is distorted. The 58-year-old woman presented with dyspepsia. No focal lesion was seen at endoscopy but there did appear to be some distortion of the mucosa of the antrum. Multiple biopsies were taken and they showed evidence of carcinoma. Examination of the resected specimen following partial gastrectomy showed an extensive carcinoma of the gastric antrum limited to the mucosa (Nolan 1978)

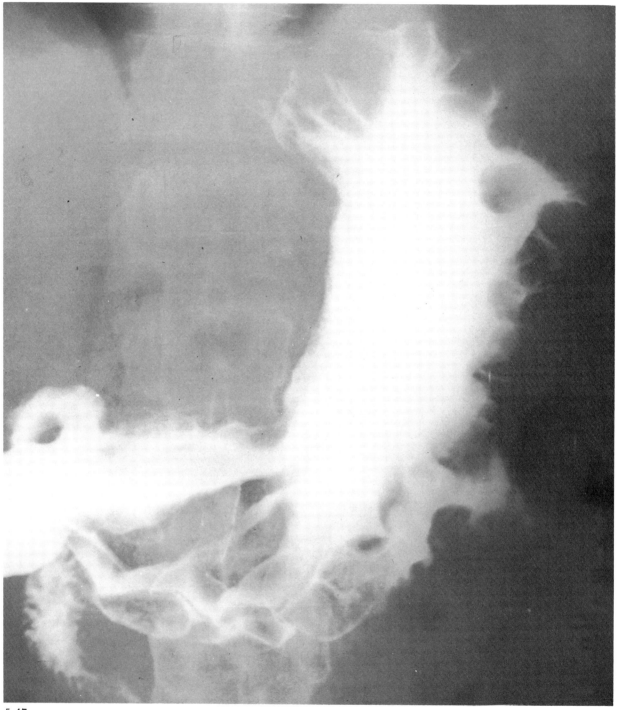

5.47

5.47 **Lymphoma** Polypoid mucosal fold thickening involving the whole stomach is seen in a female patient with established gastric lymphoma (Privett *et al.* 1977)

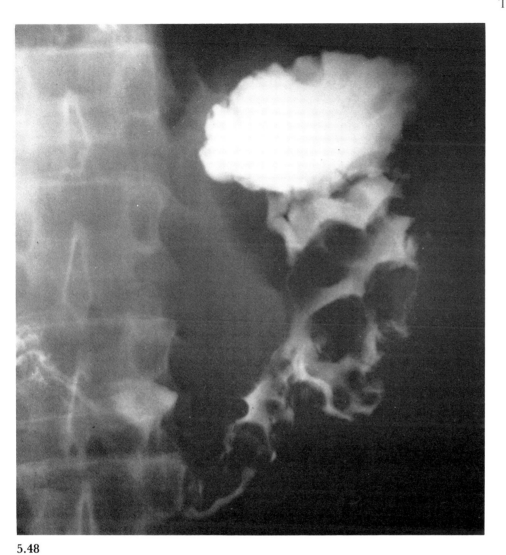

5.48

5.48 **Lymphoma** Polypoid filling defects, best seen in the body of the stomach, are shown in a man with gastric lymphoma. (Courtesy of Dr. J.T.J. Privett)

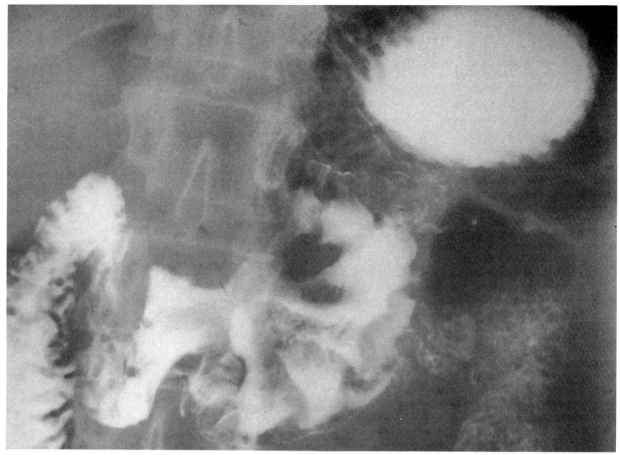

5.49

5.49 Lymphoma A gastric ulcer with radiating thickened mucosal folds is seen in a male patient with gastric lymphoma (Privett *et al*. 1977)

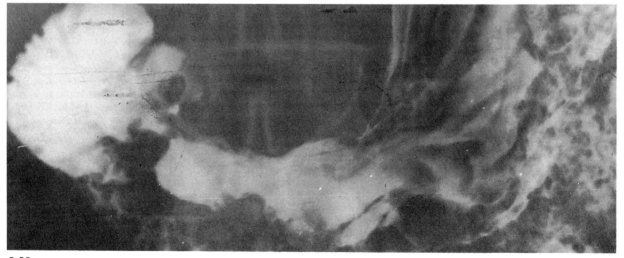

5.50

5.50 Lymphoma There is an infiltrating lesion causing narrowing and irregularity of the antrum, pylorus and the base of the duodenal cap. (Courtesy of Dr. J.T.J. Privett)

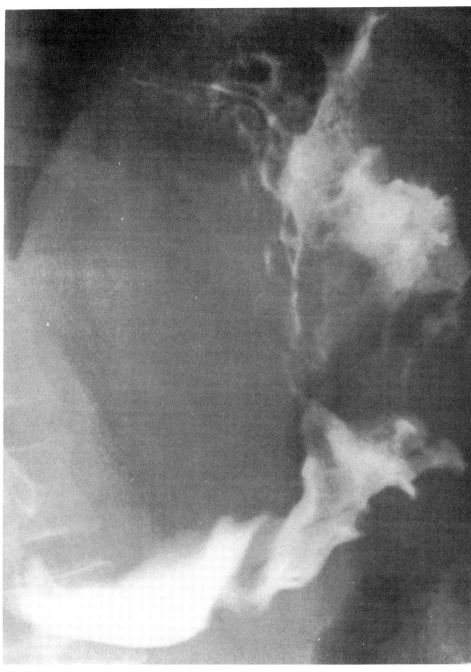

5.51

5.51 **Metastasis from malignant melanoma** A large filling defect is seen in the body of the stomach of a 31-year-old man who presented with malaise, anorexia and weight loss associated with epigastric discomfort. The patient had an axillary mass excised seven months before; the histology had shown malignant melanoma although no primary site had been found at laparotomy. At a second laparotomy, following this barium examination, a large gastric mass and a jejunal tumour were resected. Histology of the tumours showed non-pigmented melanoma. The patient died shortly afterwards from an intra-abdominal haemorrhage; metastatic melanoma were found in the brain, lung and jejunum at autopsy (Beckly 1974)

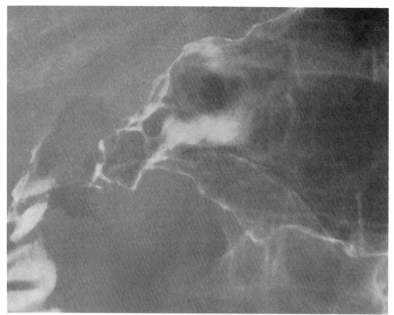

5.52

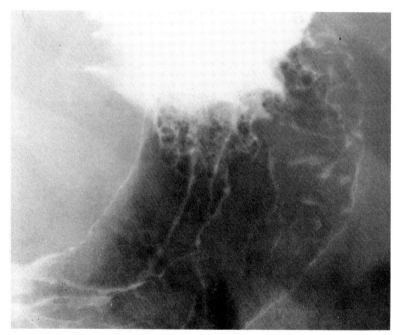

5.53

5.52 **Carcinoma of the pancreas involving the stomach** There is an infiltrating lesion seen causing distortion and narrowing of the prepyloric antrum and duodenal cap. The lesion is also displacing the greater-curve aspect of the gastric antrum upwards. The 64-year-old woman presented with nausea, anorexia, vomiting and weight loss. A carcinoma of the pancreas involving the omentum and stomach was found at operation

5.53 **Acute pancreatitis** There is gross thickening and distortion of the mucosal folds throughout the stomach in a 54-year-old man who was admitted with acute abdominal pain. He proved to have acute pancreatitis with pseudocyst formation

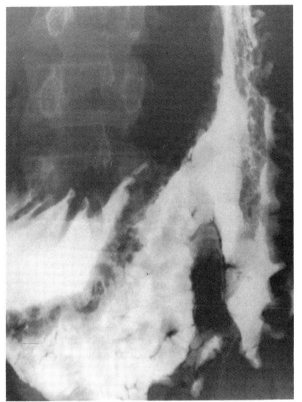

5.54a

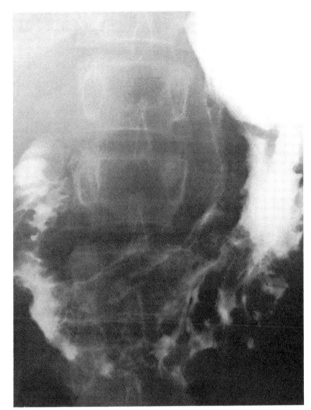

5.54b

5.54 **Menetrier's disease** There
is marked mucosal fold enlargement
of the body and proximal part of
the antrum in a 42-year-old man
who presented with a four-week
history of severe abdominal pain.
The diagnosis of.Menetrier's disease
was made on the basis of a full-
thickness biopsy obtained at
laparotomy

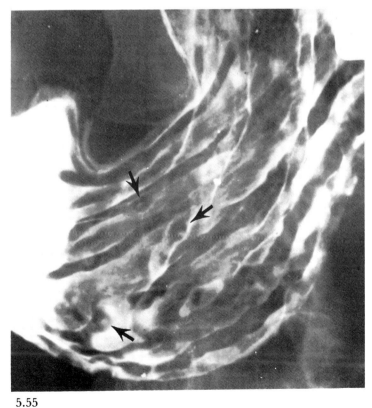

5.55 **Early Crohn's disease** A
number of aphthoid ulcers (arrows)
are demonstrated on a *double-contrast
study* of this otherwise normal stomach.
Endoscopic biopsies of the ulcers
showed changes consistent with
Crohn's disease (Kelvin & Gedgaudas
1981)

5.55

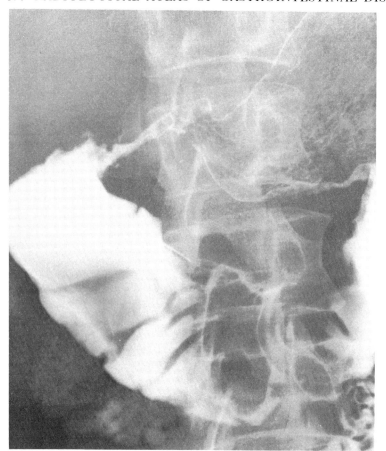

5.56

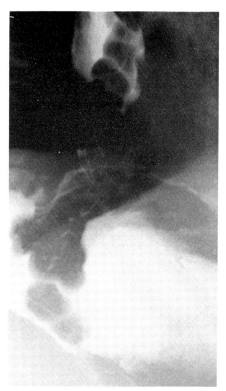

5.57a

5.56 **Crohn's disease** Gastroduodenal Crohn's
disease is causing narrowing of the antrum and
duodenal cap, giving the 'pseudo post-Billroth I'
appearance. The 32-year-old woman presented
with symptoms and signs of pyloric obstruction.
Crohn's disease involving the stomach, duodenum
and small intestine was found at operation

5.57 **Varices** a Varices are seen in the lower
oesophagus and in the fundus of the stomach.
b On this view the gastric varices are seen as
polypoid filling defects at the cardia. The 62-
year-old woman with cirrhosis was admitted to
hospital on a number of occasions with upper
gastrointestinal bleeding from varices

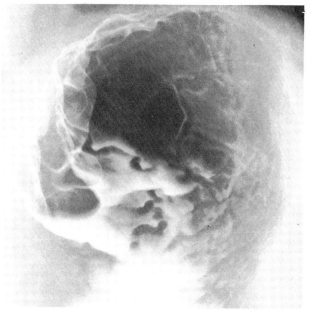

5.57b

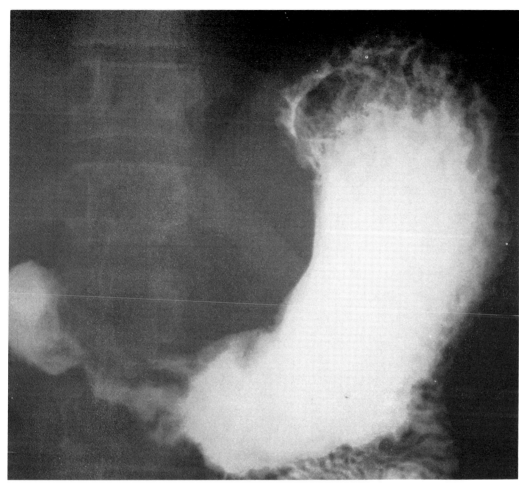

5.58a

5.58 **Syphilis** a,b There is irregularity and narrowing of the prepyloric gastric antrum with gross distortion and irregularity of the mucosal folds. (Courtesy of Dr. Leon Love)

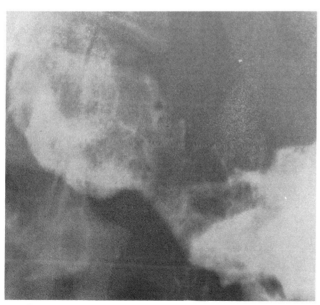

5.58b

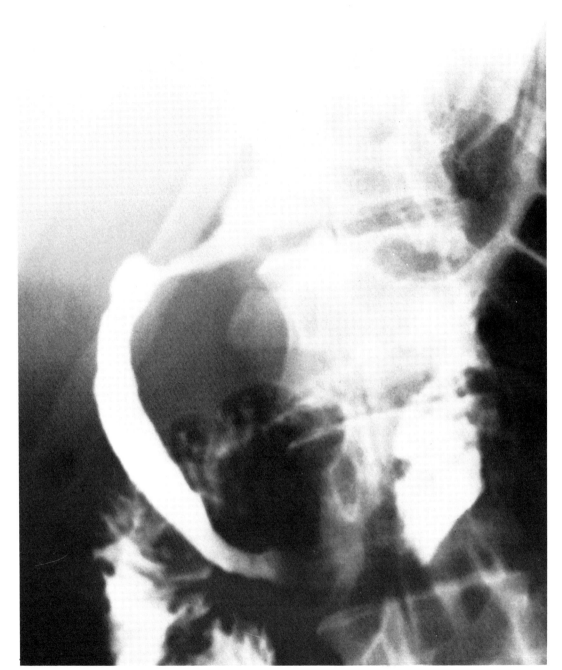

5.59

5.59 **Corrosive damage** There is considerable narrowing and shortening of the gastric antrum. The duodenal loop is also involved and is considerably narrowed. Same case as Figure 4.16. (Courtesy of Dr. Stuart Field)

6 The Duodenum

Duodenal ulceration

Benign peptic ulceration is by far the most common disease of the duodenum and the duodenal cap is the usual site of involvement. It occurs more often in males and is usually a chronic disease with recurrent exacerbations and remissions. The complications of duodenal ulceration are bleeding, perforation and obstruction. Ulceration of the duodenum distal to the cap, so-called post-bulbar ulceration, is uncommon and may have a variety of causes such as benign peptic ulceration, the Zollinger–Ellison syndrome, primary carcinoma of the duodenum, extension into the duodenum of a malignant process in an adjacent organ, or ulcerating metastases. The Zollinger–Ellison syndrome is a condition characterized by peptic and jejunal ulceration due to gastrin-secreting non-beta-cell adenomas of the pancreas causing marked hypersecretion and hyperacidity (Zollinger & Ellison 1955).

The double-contrast barium meal is an accurate method for detecting duodenal ulcers. In a study comparing the accuracy of double-contrast radiology and endoscopy in patients having elective surgery for chronic duodenal ulceration, Brown *et al.* (1978) found both methods were accurate. Endoscopy was slightly more accurate in that the surgical diagnosis correlated with endoscopy in 88 per cent of cases compared to radiology in 82 per cent. However, when both techniques were used an accuracy of 96 per cent was achieved. The barium study has the advantages that it is simple, quick to perform, it causes less patient discomfort and is associated with fewer complications than endoscopy. It should always be the initial diagnostic procedure in the investigation of suspected duodenal ulceration.

Duodenal ulcers are shown on double-contrast views as sharply defined, constant collections of barium. The duodenal cap may also be deformed although fairly large ulcers can be present without deformity of the cap. Previous ulceration may of course have deformed the duodenal cap. Anterior wall ulcers may look like ring shadows as a result of the barium dropping from the centre of the crater. In patients who have recently been bleeding from a duodenal ulcer, a small blood clot—'Berg's nodule'—may be seen in the crater.

Water-soluble contrast medium, preferably introduced into the stomach through a nasogastric tube, is used to examine patients with suspected duodenal ulcer perforation. Duodenal obstruction due to chronic peptic ulceration shows changes on barium examination similar to and often indistinguishable from pyloric stenosis.

Tumours

Benign tumours Benign tumours of the duodenum are mostly incidental findings, although they sometimes cause bleeding or obstruction. Brunner's gland hyperplasia, leiomyomas, tubular adenomas, villous adenomas, lipomas, neurogenic tumours, hamartomas, carcinoid tumours and benign tumours of the papilla of Vater are the types of benign tumour that may be found in the duodenum. Single or multiple polypoid lesions in the duodenal cap and proximal second part of the duodenum occur in Brunner's gland hyperplasia. Barium examination shows a typical cobblestone pattern which is characteristic for the condition. Nodular lymphoid hyperplasia also shows a characteristic appearance of multiple small round filling defects similar to that seen in other affected parts of the intestine. The remaining benign tumours are shown on barium studies as round or slightly lobulated well-defined filling defects. Sometimes a small area of ulceration or cavitation occurs particularly with leiomyomas. Villous adenomas normally show a villous pattern and like tubular adenomas may develop into carcinomas. Food particles in the duodenum may mimic polyps.

Carcinoma Primary carcinoma of the duodenum is uncommon, with carcinoma of the ampulla of Vater the type most frequently encountered. Jaundice, often intermittent in the early stages, is the usual presenting feature of carcinoma of the ampulla of Vater. The tumour is shown at duodenography as a rounded irregular defect occupying the medial aspect of the mid descending duodenum. Most non-ampullary carcinomas are found in the infra-ampullary part of the duodenum (Sakker & Ware 1973) with a small number occurring in the supra-ampullary part of the descending duodenum. Primary carcinoma rarely if ever involves the duodenal bulb. The presenting clinical symptoms are non-specific and include epigastric pain, bleeding and weight loss (Craig 1969; Ring & Beckly 1981). Some patients present with vomiting resulting from duodenal obstruction. The radiological appearances are shown on barium studies as infiltrating, polypoid or ulcerating lesions, similar to those of carcinoma elsewhere in the intestine (Bosse & Neely 1969).

Malignant infiltration and metastases Carcinoma of the head of the pancreas is a fairly common condition that frequently causes radiological changes in the duodenal loop. Changes may be noticed in the mucosal folds, particularly on the inner aspect of the loop. Malignant enlargement of the head of the pancreas may cause widening of the duodenal loop, irregularity of the inner border and a double contour pattern. The reversed '3' sign of Frostberg or ulceration is seen occasionally. Carcinoma of the body and tail of the pancreas frequently displaces the third and fourth parts of the duodenum causing an impression defect and splaying of the mucosal folds. A small number of patients with carcinoma of the body and tail of the pancreas may have signs of invasion of the

duodenum with mucosal destruction (Mani et al. 1966).

Since the introduction of imaging techniques, barium studies no longer play a major role in the diagnosis of carcinoma of the pancreas. However, hypotonic duodenography is particularly useful when it is performed immediately following fine-needle percutaneous cholangiography (Gourtsoyiannis & Nolan 1979).

Carcinoma of the right half of the colon and in particular carcinoma of the hepatic flexure can distort and invade the duodenal loop (Treitel et al. 1970; Veen et al. 1976). Presenting symptoms include abdominal pain, anorexia, weight loss, vomiting and bleeding; an epigastric mass may be palpable. Barium studies show loss of the normal mucosal pattern of the duodenum with infiltration causing stricturing and ulceration. Polypoid masses are occasionally seen. Duodenocolic fistula may develop due to infiltrating adenocarcinoma of the hepatic flexure (Medhurst 1956).

The duodenum can be invaded by direct spread from carcinoma of the gallbladder or right kidney. Mesenteric fibrosis due to carcinoid tumour may spread to involve the duodenal loop, and the resulting infiltration may cause narrowing and obstruction of the lumen.

Metastatic disease of the duodenum may occur secondary to malignancy elsewhere such as malignant melanoma (Beckly 1974), carcinoma of the uterus (Veen et al. 1976) and carcinoma of the kidney (Lawson et al. 1966).

Lymphomas Primary duodenal lymphomas are rare. When they are encountered the radiological appearance is similar to that of those found in the jejunum and ileum. Gastric lymphoma may spread across the pylorus into the duodenum or the duodenum may be involved with fistula from lymphomas of the small intestine (Craig & Gregson 1981).

Pancreatitis
Duodenal ileus resulting from acute pancreatitis may be seen on plain radiographs; barium studies of the duodenum show mucosal oedema, evidence of pancreatic enlargement, or enlargement of the papilla of Vater. Hypotonic duodenography demonstrates radiological changes in 64–80 per cent of patients with chronic pancreatitis (Eaton & Ferrucci 1973). There may be smooth effacement of the mucosal folds of the inner margin of the second part of the duodenum, or a serrated spiculated appearance of the inner margin and enlargement of the papilla. The appearances are non-specific and

6.1 **Duodenal ulceration** A moderate-sized ulcer crater is shown on the inferior wall of the duodenal cap. The patient, a 64-year-old man with a long history of alcohol abuse, was admitted with melaena and required an eight-unit blood transfusion. Emergency endoscopy was difficult—the endoscope did not pass into the duodenum. He was treated medically and has remained well

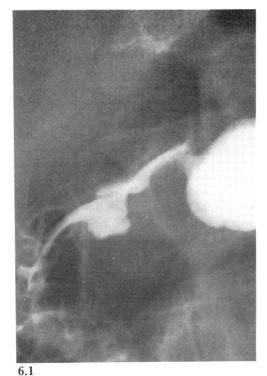

6.1

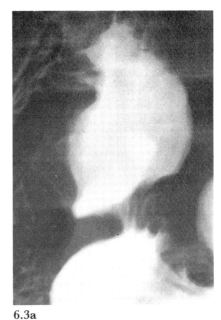

6.3a

6.2 **Duodenal ulceration** A small ulcer crater with radiating folds is seen in the base of a slightly deformed duodenal cap

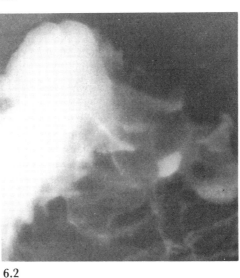

6.2

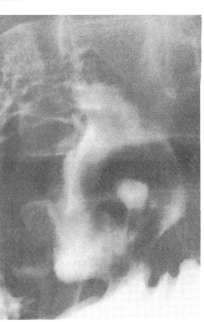

6.3b

6.3 **Duodenal ulceration** a The barium-filled duodenal cap is normal in size and shape but a central area of increased density can be identified. b Compression of the cap has expelled most of the barium and a moderate-sized ulcer crater is clearly shown. c An *oblique view* shows it is a posterior wall ulcer. The middle-aged patient was referred by her family doctor for investigation of dyspepsia of recent onset

6.4 **Duodenal ulceration** There is a small oval ulcer crater with radiating mucosal folds and moderate deformity of the duodenal cap. The 59-year-old female presented with a two-year history of dyspepsia. Endoscopy four months later found the pylorus irritable, oedematous and red and although an ulcer was not identified it was thought that one might be present beneath the oedematous folds

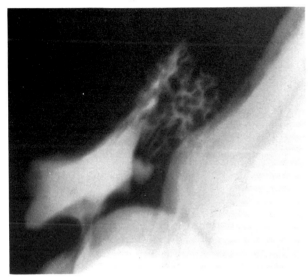

6.3c

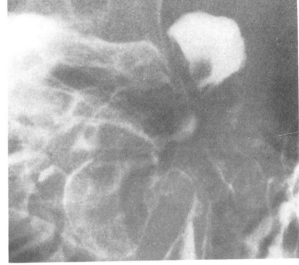

6.4

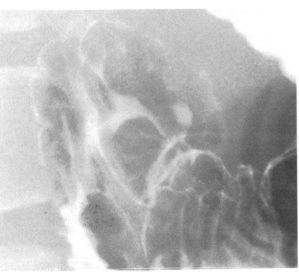

6.5

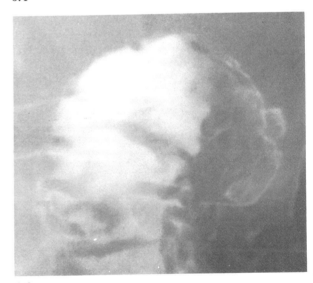

6.6

6.5 **Duodenal ulceration** The duodenal cap is slightly deformed and contains a number of mainly small ulcer craters. The patient, a 20-year-old man, presented with recurrent abdominal pain characteristic of peptic ulceration. A single-contrast barium meal two years earlier showed no abnormality. The symptoms resolved following medical treatment

6.6 **Duodenal ulceration** A moderate-sized ulcer crater is seen in the anterior wall of the duodenal cap at hypotonic duodenography. The 63-year-old man was admitted with melaena. A single-contrast examination and endoscopy found nothing to account for the bleeding. A duodenal tube was used at duodenography with a view to performing a barium study of the small intestine if the duodenum proved normal

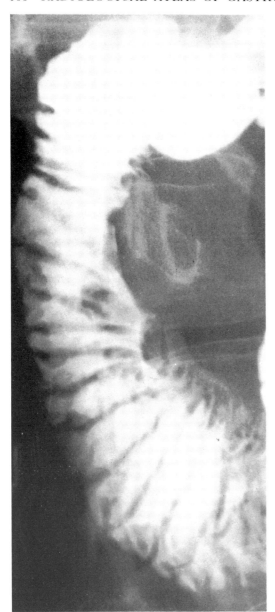

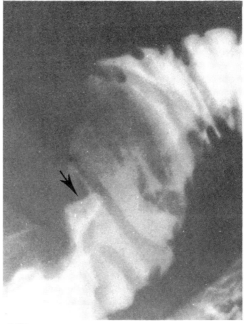

6.35

6.35 **Carcinoma of the pancreas** A lesion, infiltrating and compressing the junction of the third and fourth parts of the duodenum and with a central ulcer crater (arrow), is seen on this view obtained at the end of a barium infusion examination of the small intestine. The elderly woman was admitted with persistent gastrointestinal bleeding. Barium studies and endoscopy of the upper gastrointestinal tract and colon as well as selective visceral angiography had been performed and were negative. At operation a large carcinoma of the pancreas was found involving the third part of the duodenum

6.34

6.34 **Carcinoma of the head of the pancreas** The medial border of the second part of the duodenum is abnormal. A reversed '3' sign of Frostberg is shown with effacement and distortion of the mucosal pattern. This 75-year-old woman was admitted with obstructive jaundice. Carcinoma of the head of the pancreas was found invading the portal vein at laparotomy; a gastroenterostomy and a choledochoenterostomy were performed

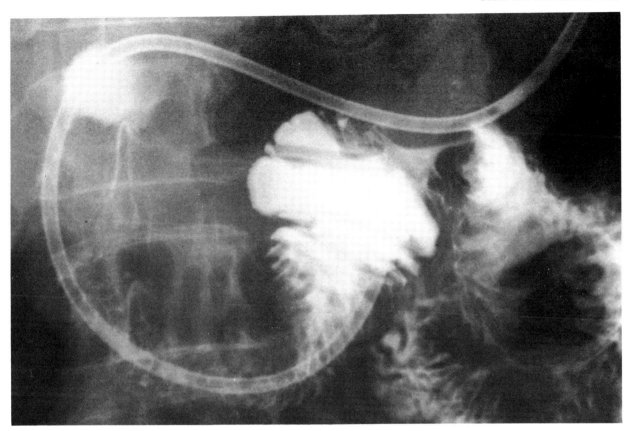

6.36a

6.36 **Carcinoma of the tail of the pancreas** a
Duodenography shows a constricting lesion obstructing
the duodenum at the ligament of Treitz. b A *spot view*
of the obstructed segment. The patient, a man in his
late sixties, was investigated because of severe vomiting
from suspected duodenal obstruction. A carcinoma of
the tail of the pancreas was found infiltrating the distal
part of the duodenum at operation

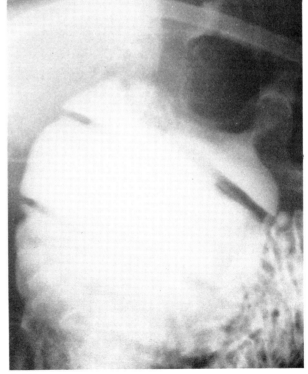

6.36b

6.37 **Carcinoma of the colon with
duodenocolic fistula** An irregular
infiltrating mass in the hepatic flexure of
the colon is outlined with barium that has
passed through a fistula from the upper
end of the second part of the duodenum.
The 84-year-old man was admitted with
faeculent vomiting. He had been
investigated ten months before for
anaemia; a barium enema at that time
showed a carcinoma of the hepatic flexure
but the patient refused surgery

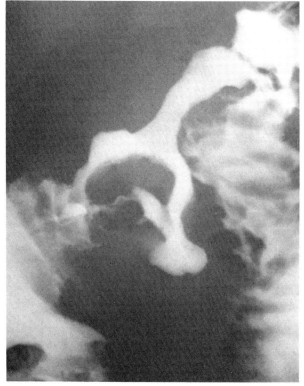

6.37

6.38 **Carcinoma of the colon infiltrating the
duodenum** Considerable infiltration and distortion of the
mucosal pattern of the second part of the duodenum is seen in
association with an ulcer crater. The 72-year-old patient was
admitted with haematemesis and melaena. She had been
operated on five months before for a carcinoma of the
ascending colon which was invading the duodenum; the part of
the tumour adherent to the duodenum could not be resected

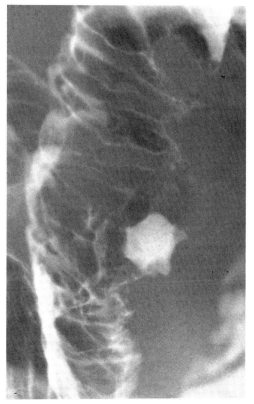

6.38

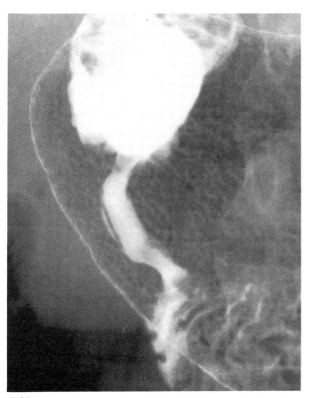

6.39

6.39 **Carcinoma of the colon infiltrating the duodenum** An infiltrating lesion is seen causing marked symmetrical narrowing of the second part of the duodenum with destruction of the mucosal pattern. The patient presented with right upper quadrant pain. Carcinoma in an inverted caecum was found involving the duodenum at operation. Same case as Figure 8.18

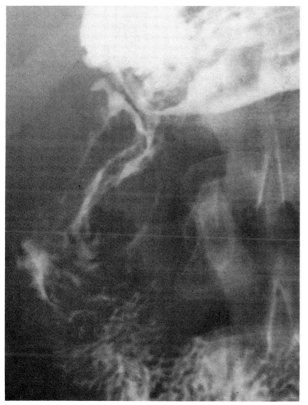

6.40

6.40 **Carcinoma of the kidney infiltrating the duodenum** The normal mucosal pattern of the proximal second part of the duodenum is destroyed and there is also marked distortion and narrowing of the lumen. The patient presented with haematemesis and a large renal mass. The diagnosis of carcinoma of the right kidney involving the duodenum was confirmed at laparotomy. (Courtesy of Dr. Shirley Roberts)

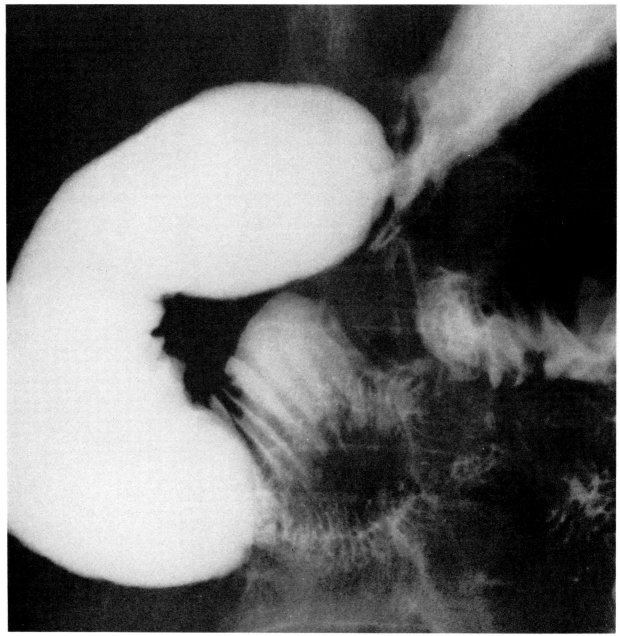

6.41

6.41 **Carcinoid tumour infiltrating the duodenum** There is distortion and destruction of the mucosal folds; narrowing of the lumen of the third and fourth parts of the duodenum is seen causing some degree of obstruction. This view of the duodenum was taken during a barium infusion examination of the small intestine. Extensive infiltration of most of the small intestine was shown. The 70-year-old female patient, with the carcinoid syndrome and known widespread metastatic carcinoid tumour from a primary tumour in the ileum, was admitted to hospital for assessment

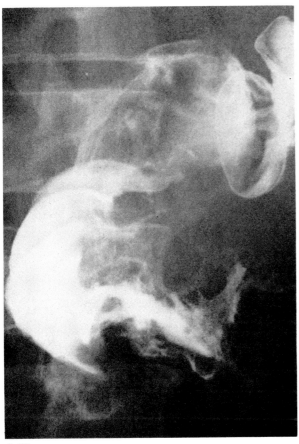

6.42

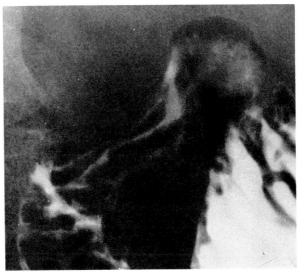

6.43

6.42 **Duodenal lymphoma** Extensive infiltration of the duodenum is seen with destruction of the mucosal pattern, narrowing of the lumen and considerable distortion. The 49-year-old man was admitted with vomiting. Eight months earlier a non-Hodgkin's lymphoma involving the head of the pancreas was found at laparotomy. (Courtesy of Dr. Michael C. Collins)

6.43 **Pancreatitis** Mucosal oedema is shown at the junction of the first and second parts of the duodenum. The 35-year-old man with a history of alcohol abuse was admitted after a long bout of heavy drinking with severe abdominal pain, haematemesis and melaena. Oesophageal varices, shown on the barium examination and endoscopy, were the presumed site of bleeding. The changes shown here and the severe abdominal pain would indicate that the patient also had pancreatitis

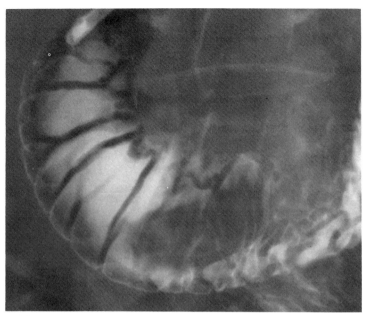

6.44

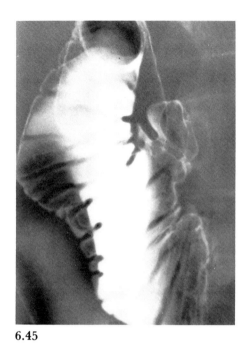

6.45

6.44 **Chronic pancreatitis** *Hypotonic duodenography* shows a slightly enlarged papilla of Vater, irregularity of the mucosal pattern of the inner border and partial compression of the third part of the duodenum. The middle-aged woman, with a history of alcohol abuse, developed duodenal obstruction four months later requiring laparotomy. There was enlargement of the head of the pancreas and a mass that was not hard. Biopsies obtained showed no evidence of malignancy and the diagnosis of chronic pancreatitis was confirmed

6.45 **Duodenal diverticulum** A diverticulum is seen in the mid second part of the duodenum

6.46 **Duodenal diverticulum** A large diverticulum is seen extending upwards from the third part of the duodenum

6.47 **Crohn's disease of the duodenal cap** There is a cobblestone pattern and some erosions in the proximal half of the duodenal cap. The patient previously had two resections of the small intestine for Crohn's disease (Nolan 1981)

6.48 **Crohn's disease** The duodenal cap is deformed and there is loss of the mucosal pattern in the second part of the duodenum. Shortening of the proximal second part of the duodenum and a couple of erosions in the prepyloric antrum are also seen. Four months before, this 26-year-old man had a laparotomy for a suspected duodenal ulcer when the duodenal wall was found to be thickened and an ulcer was excised. The adjacent duodenum showed histological appearances consistent with Crohn's disease

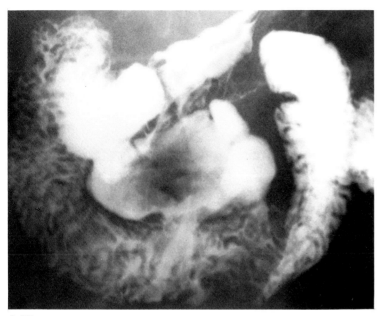

6.46

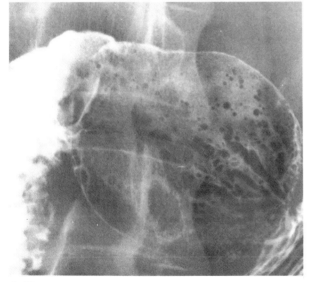

6.47

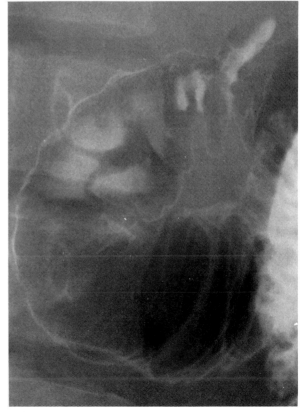

6.48

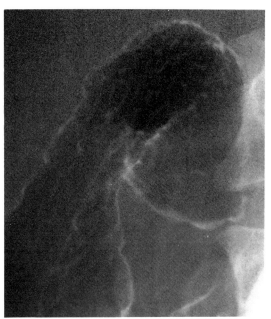

6.49 **Crohn's disease** a A *double-contrast view* shows a cobblestone pattern in the duodenal cap and the proximal descending duodenum. b The distal descending duodenum is relatively spared but there is marked involvement of the third and fourth parts with stricture formation (arrows). The patient who was known to have Crohn's disease of the duodenum and ileum was admitted with abdominal pain and vomiting

6.49a

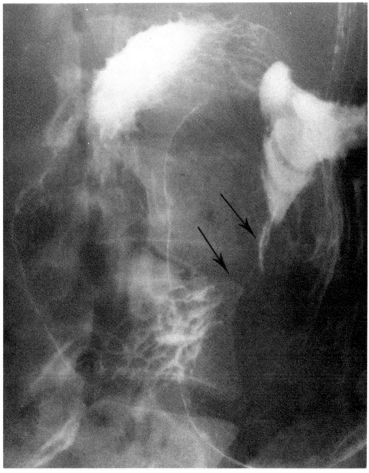

6.49b

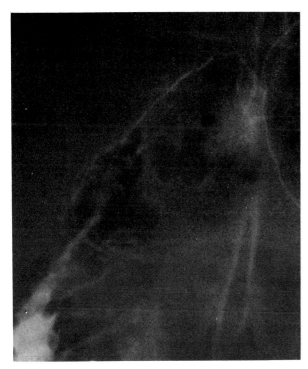

6.50

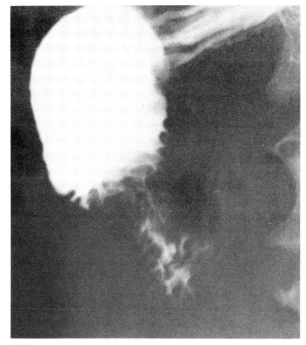

6.51a

6.50 **Duodenal varix** A lobulated filling defect characteristic of a varix is seen in the duodenal cap. The 33-year-old man was admitted following an episode of severe melaena. He had a long history of extrahepatic portal hypertension following neonatal umbilical sepsis and 18 years before had a proximal gastrectomy and splenectomy. Extensive oesophageal and gastric varices were also seen. Occlusion of the portal vein was confirmed at angiography. A mesocaval anastomosis was performed and he remains well three years later

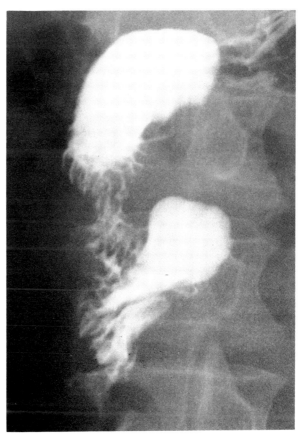

6.51b

6.51 **Intramural haematoma** a An extrinsic compression defect in the second part of the duodenum is causing considerable narrowing of the lumen and delay in the passage of barium. b On a view taken a short time later a small amount of barium has passed the narrowed site and the mucosa of the narrowed segment is shown intact. This 60-year-old man with suspected myocardial infarction had been treated with anticoagulants four days before. When the diagnosis was not confirmed the treatment was stopped and he was discharged from hospital. He developed persistent vomiting and was re-admitted. At laparotomy the diagnosis of intramural haematoma was confirmed and a gastroenterostomy was performed

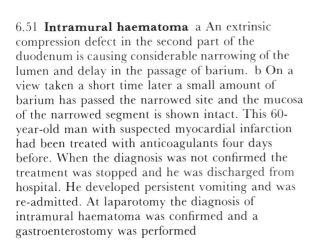

7 The Small Intestine

Crohn's disease

Crohn's disease is a chronic granulomatous disease of unknown aetiology which mainly affects young adults. Any part of the gastrointestinal tract may be involved but the small intestine is the principal site. The ileum, particularly the terminal ileum, is the part of the intestine most frequently involved. Disease of the terminal ileum is often present in continuity with Crohn's disease of the caecum or of the caecum and ascending colon. The extent of small intestine involved varies considerably from less than 1 cm to very extensive involvement.

Patients with Crohn's disease present with a variety of clinical symptoms and signs. Abdominal pain and diarrhoea, often with weight loss, are presenting symptoms in the majority of patients. It is not unusual for patients to present with an 'acute abdomen' simulating appendicitis. Intestinal obstruction, fistulae, anaemia and retardation of growth are other modes of presentation of the disease.

The barium infusion is an extremely valuable examination in the diagnosis and management of Crohn's disease of the small intestine. The radiological signs of Crohn's disease of the small intestine as shown by the barium infusion can be classified as follows (Nolan 1980; Nolan & Gourtsoyiannis 1980; Nolan 1981): ulceration—discrete ulcers, fissure ulcers, longitudinal ulcers, sinuses and fistulae; cobblestoning; thickening and/or distortion of the valvulae conniventes; stenosis; dilatation proximal to stenosis; asymmetrical involvement; skip lesions; inflammatory polyps; featureless outline; thickening of the wall of the intestine; gross distortion; a mass; adhesions.

Most discrete ulcers are seen *en face* as small collections of barium, often surrounded by translucent zones due to oedema. Fissure ulcers are fairly common and are seen in profile; they are mostly short but some penetrate the wall of the intestine to a depth of 5 mm or more. These deep fissure ulcers are mostly seen in the terminal ileum or in the ileum just proximal to ileocolic anastomosis sites. Long longitudinal ulcers along the mesenteric border of the intestine are not a common finding in my experience, but they are frequently seen in Japanese patients with Crohn's disease. Sinuses, which sometimes lead to abscess cavities, are another form of ulceration that may be present. Internal fistulae between different parts of the intestinal tract, or between the intestine and other organs, or to·the skin may be seen.

The cobblestone pattern is a sign encountered fairly frequently in Crohn's disease. In most cases it is caused by a combination of longitudinal and transverse fissures separating intact portions of mucosa. In others oedematous mucosal and submucosal folds produce a cobblestone pattern (Marshak & Lindner 1976). There is often thickening and distortion of the valvulae conniventes in Crohn's disease and this is probably the earliest detectable radiological sign of small intestinal Crohn's disease in the majority of patients.

Narrowing of the lumen causing stenosis is seen frequently.

The stenotic segments may be short or long and they may be single or multiple. Dilatation of the intestine, due to chronic obstruction, is present in many patients with strictures. Strictures may, however, cause acute small intestinal obstruction without significant dilatation. The 'string sign' (Kantor 1934), which is due to spasm in diseased segments of intestine, is considered to be pathognomonic of Crohn's disease when the barium follow-through examination is used. It is not seen with the infusion examination as the narrowed segments of intestine can be filled with barium and their true calibre demonstrated.

Discontinuous involvement, shown as asymmetry and skip lesions, is a feature of Crohn's disease. Inflammatory polyps, seen as small discrete round filling defects, are occasionally present when the disease is extensive and severe. A featureless outline of the diseased intestine may be seen in Crohn's disease, but is an uncommon finding. There may be evidence of thickening of the wall of the diseased intestine, as shown by displacement of the adjacent barium-filled loops of intestine. Gross distortion of the involved intestine may be seen in the distal ileum when the disease is complicated by abscess and fistula formation. Occasionally a large abscess develops and may be shown radiologically as a mass in the right iliac fossa displacing the adjacent loops of intestine. Adhesions may develop between diseased and normal segments or between a number of diseased segments of intestine.

Idiopathic chronic ulcerative enteritis

Idiopathic chronic ulcerative enteritis is a rare condition of unknown aetiology where malabsorption is associated with non-specific ulceration of the small intestine (Mills *et al.* 1980). The disease presents as a chronic illness characterized by diarrhoea, weight loss and steatorrhoea. The jejunum is the site most frequently involved. Intestinal obstruction, perforation and haemorrhage supervene causing a high mortality rate. Barium examination shows multiple separate strictures of the small intestine with ulceration, dilatation and pseudodiverticulum formation.

Infections and infestations

Tuberculosis Intestinal tuberculosis is rare in Britain, North America and many of the industrialized countries where the incidence of Crohn's disease is high. It is not uncommon in tropical countries and in Britain is mostly seen in patients who come from areas of the world where the disease is endemic.

The radiological appearances of tuberculosis of the small intestine are similar to Crohn's disease and like Crohn's disease the ileocaecal area is the most common site of involvement. There are features of the radiological appearances which help to distinguish tuberculosis from Crohn's disease. Free perforation is not uncommon in tuberculosis but is rare in Crohn's disease (Vaidya & Sodhi 1978). Many patients with tuberculosis of the small intestine present initially with acute obstruction whereas this is uncommon in Crohn's disease. In ileocaecal tuberculosis the segment of terminal ileum involved is normally shorter than in Crohn's disease (Brombart *et al.* 1961).

Asymmetry in Crohn's disease, when present, helps differentiate it from tuberculosis (Bodart *et al.* 1961). Cobblestoning is a feature of Crohn's disease which is not seen in tuberculosis (Morson & Dawson 1979). Longitudinal ulcers are frequently seen in Crohn's disease in Japan and were seen in 82 per cent of cases reported by Yamagata *et al.* (1979). They are not seen in tuberculosis and the Japanese consider it a very useful sign in differentiating Crohn's disease from tuberculosis.

***Yersinia* infections** Acute inflammation of the terminal ileum is a feature of infection with *Yersinia enterocolitica* and *Yersinia pseudotuberculosis*. Right iliac fossa pain and diarrhoea are the presenting clinical features. At laparotomy the terminal ileum and caecum show gross hyperaemic swelling and oedema together with massive enlargement of the lymph nodes. Radiologically the changes are limited to the terminal 20 cm of ileum (van Wiechen 1974). The mucosal folds show a tortuous course, are increased in number and are unmistakably broadened. Small filling defects due to lymphoid hyperplasia are also seen and there is thickening of the wall of the terminal ileum.

Giardiasis *Giardia lamblia*, a flagellate protozoan parasite of the upper small intestine, is commonly associated with symptomatic disease in man (Wright *et al.* 1977). In Britain giardiasis is nearly always seen in people who have travelled abroad. The most common symptoms are abdominal pain, diarrhoea, lassitude and weight loss. On barium studies non-specific thickening of the mucosal folds of the distal duodenum and proximal jejunum is seen. Stool examination may be insufficient to exclude the diagnosis and small intestine aspiration may be necessary to demonstrate the parasite.

Strongyloidiasis *Strongyloides stercoralis* is an intestinal nemotode and individuals infected with it are often asymptomatic. They may have abdominal pain, nausea and vomiting, weight loss and

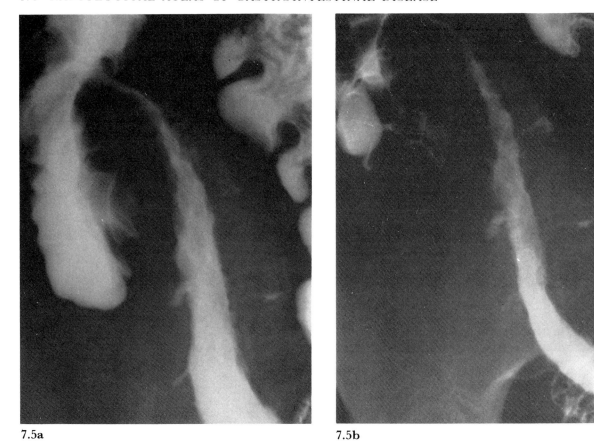

7.5a   7.5b

7.5 **Fissure ulcers and subserosal abscesses in Crohn's disease** a,b There is severe involvement of the terminal ileum. The wall of the diseased intestine is markedly thickened and a number of deep fissure ulcers are seen. Collections of barium are present in small abscess cavities deep in the fissure ulcers. The patient, a 19-year-old female, presented with abdominal pain and diarrhoea. Crohn's disease was diagnosed on the basis of this examination and medical treatment commenced. Two months later the patient's condition deteriorated and at an emergency laparotomy a large abscess was found. Examination of the resected specimen confirmed the presence of deep fissure ulcers and small subserosal abscesses (Nolan & Piris 1980)

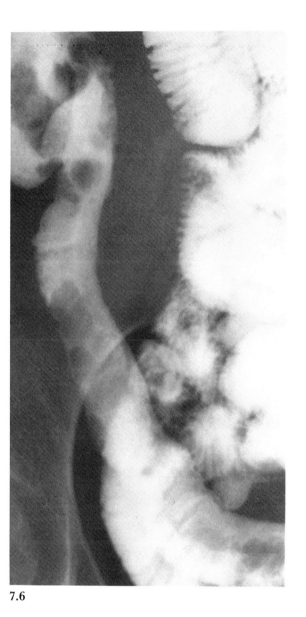

7.6

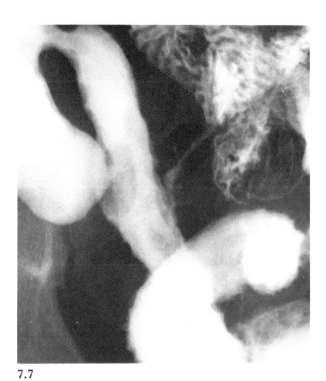

7.7

7.7 **Sinus track in Crohn's disease** A sinus track
passing medially from the ileum is outlined with
barium in a 23-year-old man with ileocaecal
Crohn's disease (Nolan & Gourtsoyiannis 1980)

7.6 **Longitudinal ulcer in Crohn's disease** A
long longitudinal ulcer, 20 cm long and about 6 mm
deep, is seen on the mesenteric border of the
terminal ileum in an 18-year-old female with a five-
year history of Crohn's disease

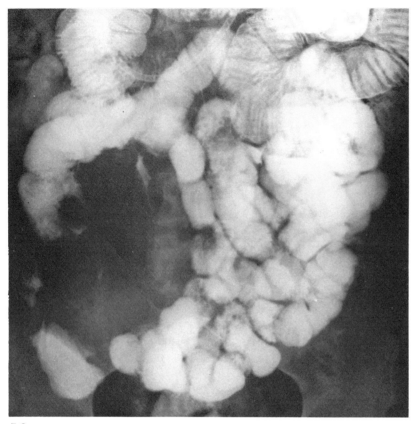

7.8a

7.8 Mass and sinus track in Crohn's disease a A large mass is seen displacing adjacent ileum, caecum and ascending colon. There is poor filling of the terminal ileum due to compression from the mass and spasm. b On this view part of the distal ileum has filled with barium but poor filling of the terminal ileum persists. A thin track of barium is seen passing upwards into, but not filling, an abscess. This 24-year-old man was found to have Crohn's disease at laparotomy two years before. He presented with recurrence of symptoms and on examination had a mass in the right iliac fossa

7.9 Multiple sinuses and abscesses in Crohn's disease There is gross distortion of the ileocaecal junction and multiple sinus tracks leading to small abscess cavities. The patient, a 30-year-old man with known Crohn's disease, was admitted to hospital for the investigation of pyrexia of unknown origin

7.10 Ileoileal fistulae in Crohn's disease

7.11 Ileovesical fistula in Crohn's disease The patient, a 22-year-old man, gave a three-year history of pneumaturia and faecaluria. Excretion urography and cystography had been performed twice but on each occasion showed no abnormality. Gross distortion and narrowing of the distal ileum is seen with dilatation of a short segment of ileum proximal to the narrowed segment. Some barium has passed into the urinary bladder and slightly opaque urine outlines the bladder wall (arrow)

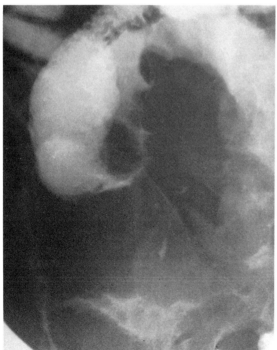

7.8b

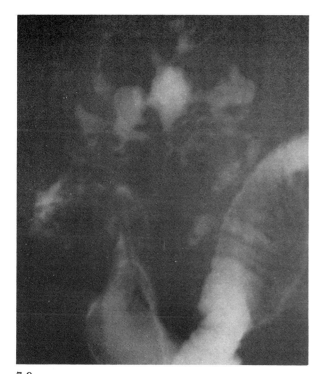

7.9

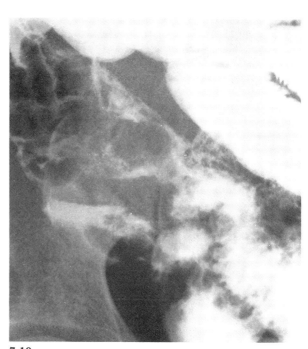

7.10

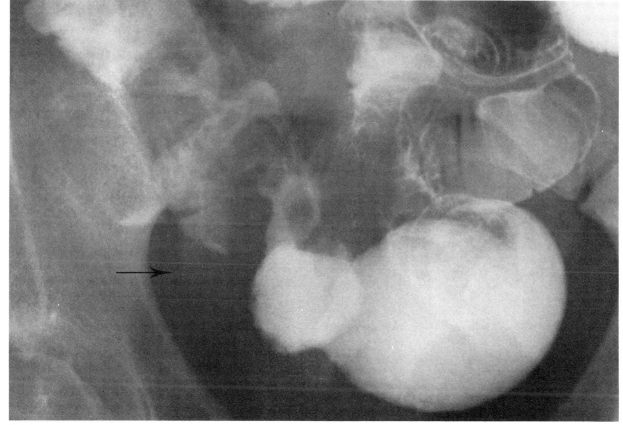

7.11

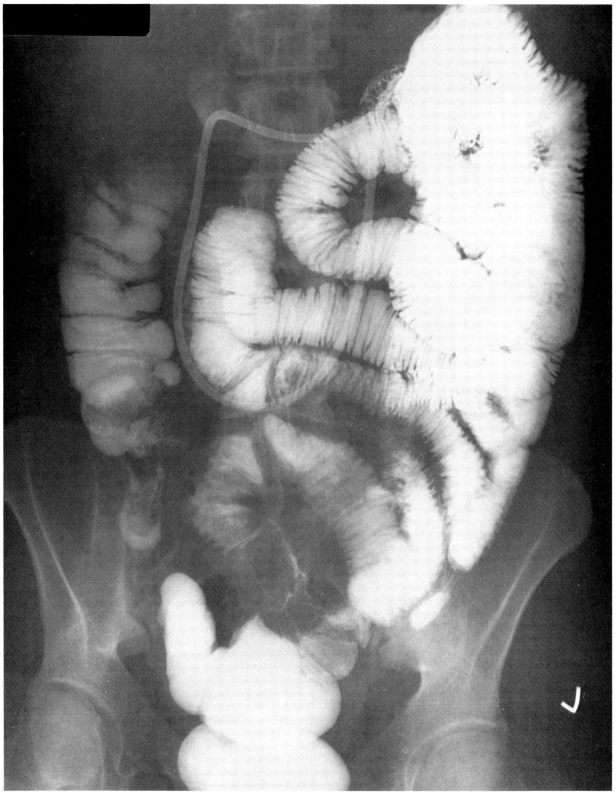

7.12

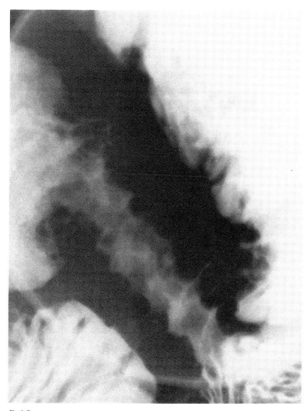

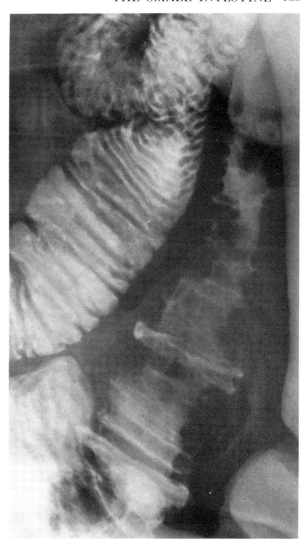

7.13

7.14

7.13 Cobblestoning and fissure ulcers in Crohn's disease
An irregular cobblestone pattern is seen proximal to the site of an ileocolic anastomosis; a number of deep fissure ulcers are also present. The 38-year-old patient had two previous resections for Crohn's disease. A barium examination six months earlier showed thickened valvulae conniventes proximal to the ileocolic anastomosis site (Nolan & Gourtsoyiannis 1980)

7.12 Ileocolic fistulae in Crohn's disease
Barium is seen passing through ileosigmoid fistulae and outlining the distal sigmoid colon and rectum before the head of the barium column has reached the transverse colon. Ileocaecal fistulae can also be identified. The 37-year-old female, with a ten-year history of Crohn's disease, was examined because of an acute exacerbation of symptoms

7.14 Thickened valvulae conniventes and cobblestoning in Crohn's disease
A 15-cm length of ileum proximal to the site of an ileocolic anastomosis shows gross thickening of the valvulae conniventes proximally, and an irregular cobblestone pattern adjacent to the anastomosis site. The patient, a 32-year-old female, had a seven-year history of Crohn's disease with three previous resections. On this occasion she was admitted because of exacerbation of symptoms; she presented with abdominal pain, diarrhoea, joint pains and perianal abscesses (Nolan 1981)

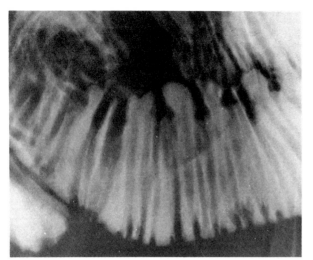

7.15

7.15 Thickened valvulae conniventes in Crohn's disease Slight thickening and irregularity of the valvulae conniventes is seen on a *spot view* of a segment of ileum in a 23-year-old man who previously had a resection of the terminal ileum for Crohn's disease

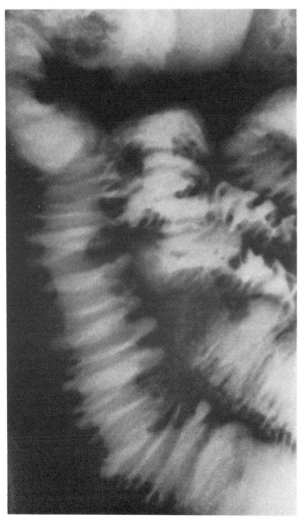

7.16

7.16 Thickened valvulae conniventes in Crohn's disease There is marked thickening of the valvulae conniventes in the ileum just proximal to the site of an ileocolic anastomosis. The 32-year-old female had four previous resections for Crohn's disease

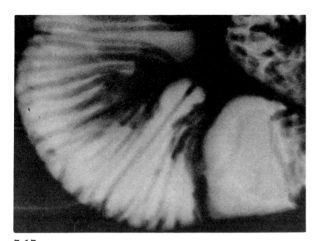

7.17

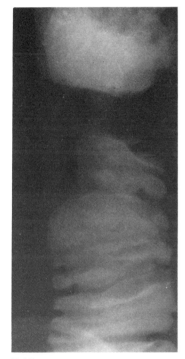

7.18

7.17 **A very short stricture in Crohn's disease** This 36-year-old man with a history of previous ileal resection had multiple Crohn's strictures throughout the small intestine

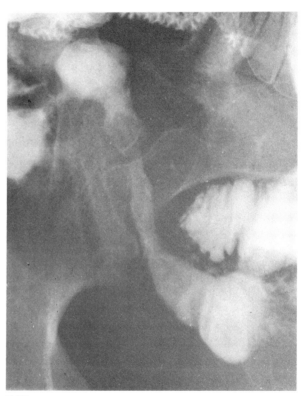

7.19

7.18 **Crohn's stricture** There is a short stricture, asymmetry and thickened folds in a segment of recurrent disease just proximal to the site of an ileocolic anastomosis in a 38-year-old female with a history of previous right hemicolectomy for Crohn's disease

7.19 **A long Crohn's stricture of the terminal ileum** This was the only view that showed the true calibre of the narrowed segment. The patient, a 27-year-old female, was found to have Crohn's disease of the terminal ileum at a previous laparotomy performed because of right iliac fossa pain (Nolan & Piris 1980)

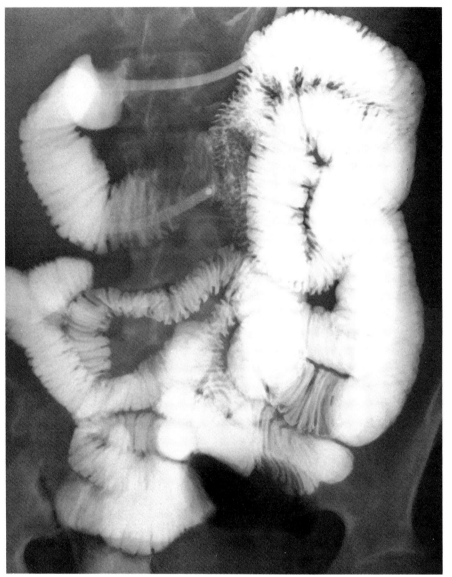

7.20a

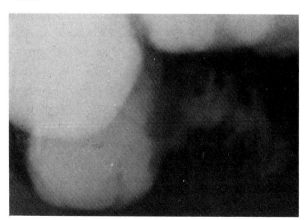

7.20b

7.20 **Short Crohn's stricture causing obstruction** The 19-year-old female was admitted with subacute small intestinal obstruction. a The jejunum and proximal ileum were normal but there is almost complete hold-up in the passage of barium through one of the pelvic loops of ileum. b An *oblique view* shows a short tight stricture. A Meckel's diverticulum with an adjacent stricture was found at operation. The remainder of the small intestine was normal. Histological examination of the resected specimen showed Crohn's disease (Nolan & Marks 1981)

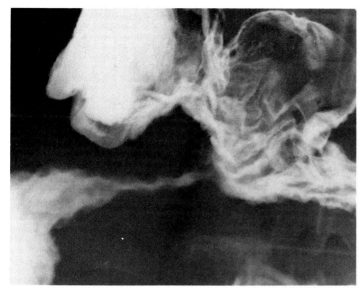

7.21 **Crohn's stricture** A stricture is seen in the ileum at the site of an end-to-side ileocolic anastomosis. The patient, a 51-year-old female, had a resection of small intestine for Crohn's disease 25 years before

7.22 **Multiple Crohn's strictures** Multiple tight strictures with segments of dilatation proximal to many of the narrowed segments are seen in the mid small intestine. The 43-year-old female was known to have had Crohn's disease for five years

7.21

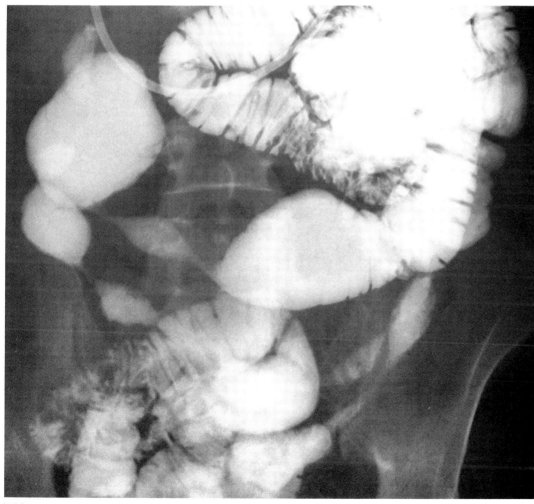

7.22

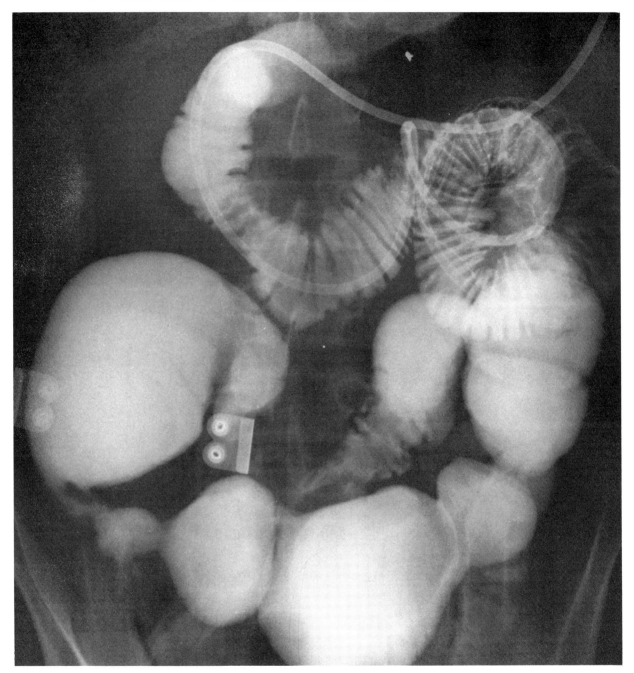

7.23

7.23 Crohn's strictures Multiple strictures with dilatation proximal to the strictures are seen in a 24-year-old man who had had a previous resection of ileum and an ileostomy for Crohn's disease

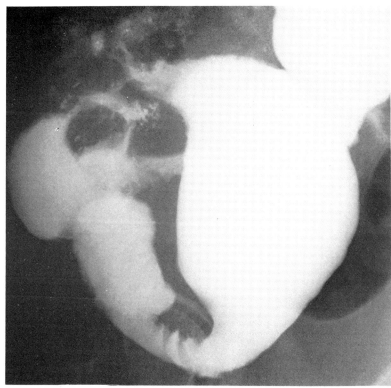

7.24

7.24 **Strictures and adhesions in Crohn's disease** This 52-year-old man previously had a resection for Crohn's disease and was admitted to hospital on this occasion with symptoms of intestinal obstruction. A number of narrowed segments with dilatation proximally are seen. At operation an inflammatory mass was found

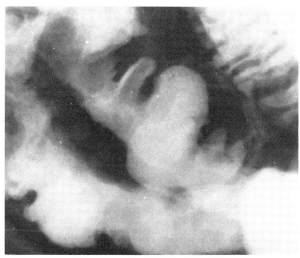

7.25

7.25 **Asymmetrical involvement in Crohn's disease** Pseudodiverticula formation has resulted from asymmetrical involvement of the distal ileum with Crohn's disease. The patient, a 57-year-old man with acromegaly, was diagnosed as having Crohn's disease at laparotomy six months before (Nolan & Piris 1980)

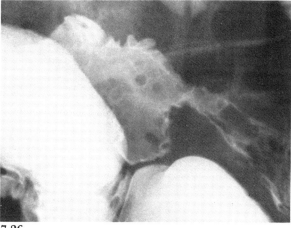

7.26

7.26 **Inflammatory polyps in Crohn's disease** Multiple small round filling defects are seen on a barium study of a 22-year-old woman with extensive Crohn's disease of the small intestine (Nolan & Piris 1980)

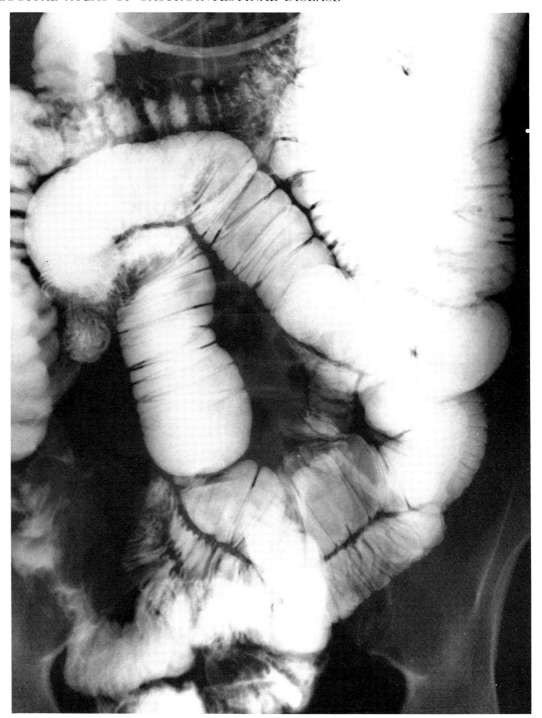

7.27a

7.27 **Skip lesions in Crohn's disease** a A short
tight stricture is seen in the ileum with slight
proximal dilatation. b Another stricture, with
asymmetry and proximal dilatation, is seen in the
terminal ileum. The strictures were separated by
normal small intestine. The 37-year-old female
presented with colicky abdominal pain and iron
deficiency anaemia but no history of diarrhoea

7.28 **Featureless outline in Crohn's
disease** The terminal ileum has a featureless
outline with narrowing of the lumen and asymmetry

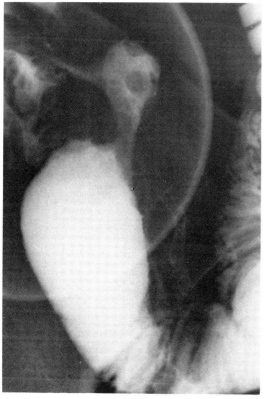

7.27b

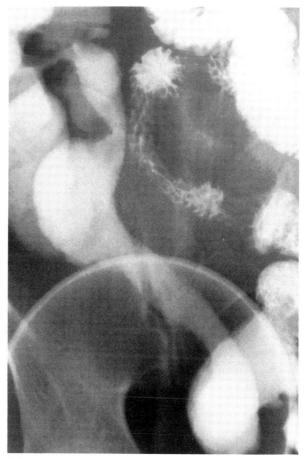

7.28

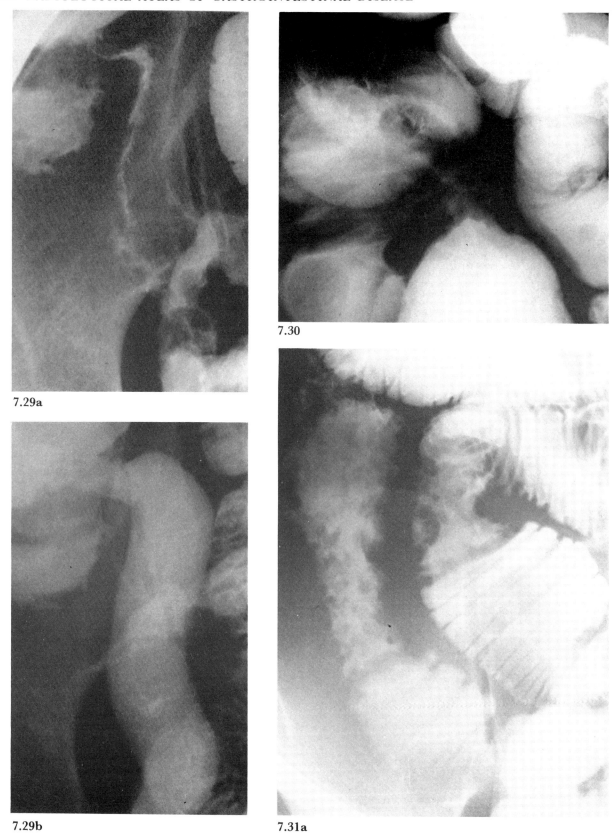

7.29a

7.30

7.29b

7.31a

7.29 The 'string sign' and a featureless outline in Crohn's disease a On this view there is spasm of the terminal ileum giving the 'string sign' appearance. b Moments later the terminal ileum has distended and is shown to be of normal calibre. There is loss of the normal mucosal pattern resulting in a smooth featureless appearance. The patient, a 51-year-old woman, had a long history of ileocolic Crohn's disease. The appearances shown here are similar to those of reflex ileitis seen sometimes in ulcerative colitis. A split ileostomy was performed because of severe colonic disease and examination of the terminal ileum showed definite evidence of involvement with Crohn's disease. This examination illustrates how unreliable the 'string sign' is in assessing the true calibre of the lumen of the small intestine

7.30 Ileocaecal tuberculosis There is a short segment of marked narrowing at the ileocaecal junction with dilatation of the more proximal ileum. The patient, a 23-year-old Indian woman, presented with intestinal obstruction. Tuberculosis was confirmed at operation

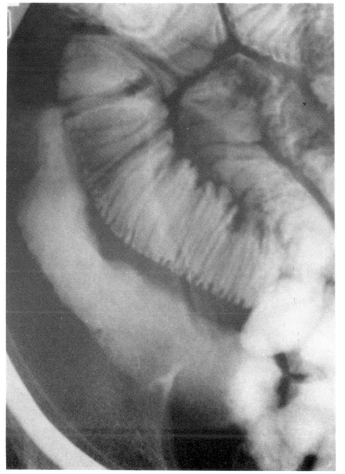

7.31 Ileal tuberculosis a Mucosal ulceration with thickening of the intestinal wall is seen involving a 10-cm segment of distal ileum. A short segment of adjacent ileum is also involved. There is an ulcer with surrounding oedema in the shorter segment adjacent to the thickened wall of the two adherent segments. The appearances would suggest that the disease spread from one segment to the other through the wall of the intestine. The patient, a 36-year-old Korean man, presented with a two-month history of nausea, anorexia, epigastric pain, weight loss and night sweats. On examination he was cachectic. A chest radiograph showed active pulmonary tuberculosis. b The ileal ulceration has healed following antituberculous chemotherapy

7.31b

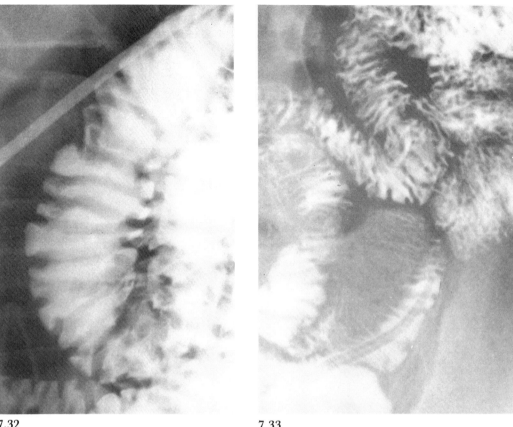

7.32

7.33

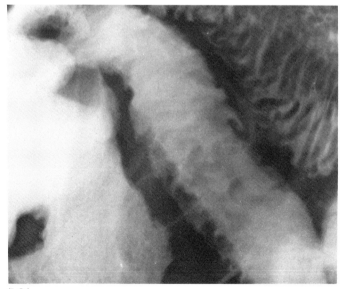

7.34

7.32 **Giardiasis** There is marked thickening of the valvulae conniventes of the proximal jejunum. The appearances are not specific for giardiasis. The patient presented with abdominal pain, diarrhoea and weight loss. A jejunal biopsy was performed because of the radiological findings, and *Giardia lambiia* were seen on examination of the biopsy specimens

7.33 **Ascariasis** A single worm is shown in the ileum and a thin track of barium can be seen outlining its alimentary tract

7.34 *Yersinia enterocolitica* **infection** The distal ileum is slightly abnormal with some thickening of the wall and the mucosal folds are increased in number, broadened and tortuous. The 36-year-old woman presented with right iliac fossa pain. The antibody titre for *Yersinia enterocolitica* was positive

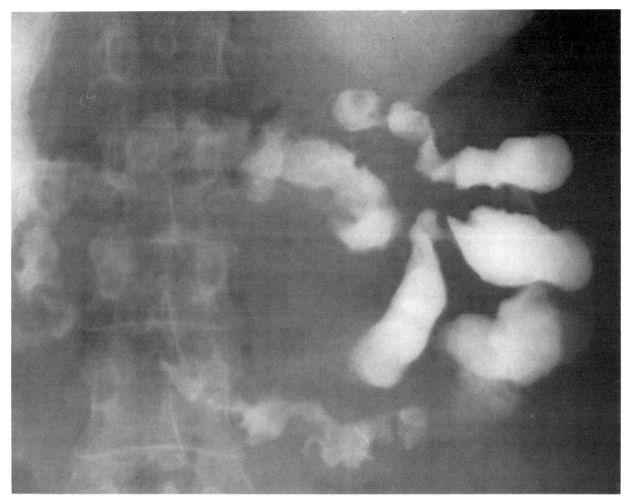

7.35

7.35 Strongyloidiasis The distal duodenum and proximal jejunum are grossly abnormal with loss of the valvulae conniventes, thickening of the wall and narrowing of the lumen; multiple strictures are causing upper gastrointestinal obstruction. The patient, a 47-year-old Jamaican, had been admitted to hospital with a subarachnoid haemorrhage and when her condition improved she complained of abdominal pain. Strongyloidiasis was suspected on the basis of this examination and *Strongyloides stercoralis* was found in fluid aspirated from the duodenum. The patient left the West Indies 16 years before. (Courtesy of Dr. J.C. MacLarnon)

7.36 **Leiomyoma** A round slightly irregular polypoid filling defect is seen projecting into the lumen of the proximal ileum on a view taken during a retrograde barium examination of the small intestine. The 50-year-old woman was investigated because of obscure gastrointestinal bleeding. A barium follow-through had failed to detect the lesion. Following resection of the tumour which proved to be a leiomyoma the patient remained well without further bleeding (Miller & Lehman 1978)

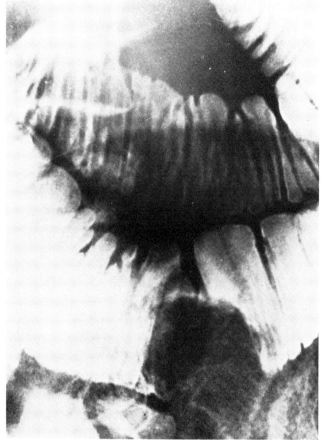

7.36

7.37 **Haemangioma** a The wall of a short segment of small intestine is distorted and irregular (arrows). b A further view of this area shows small phleboliths adjacent to the abnormal segment of intestine. c An *angiogram* of the resected specimen. The 26-year-old woman presented with melaena. Selective superior mesenteric angiography was the first investigation; no abnormal vascular pattern was demonstrated but the presence of phleboliths was noted. Following the barium study the patient was operated on and the haemangiomatous lesion was resected. (Courtesy of Dr. Louise Sheppard)

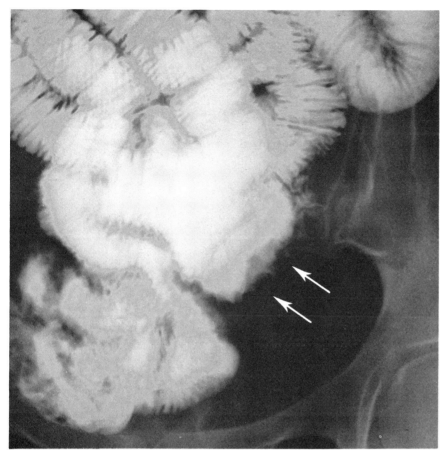

7.37a

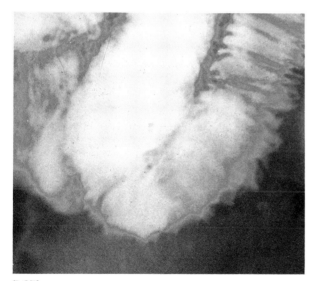

7.37b

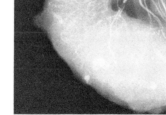

7.37c

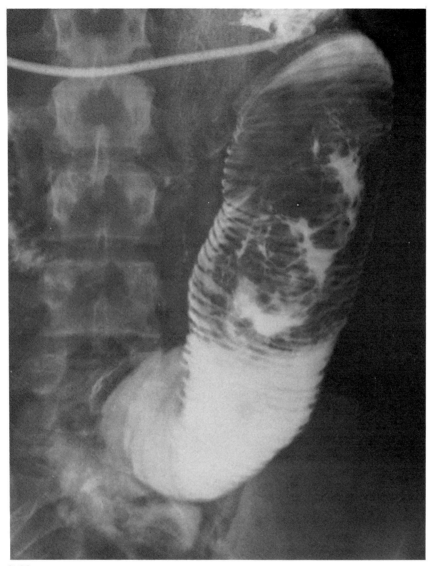

7.38

7.38 Peutz–Jeghers syndrome Two large slightly irregular polyps are shown causing jejunal intussusception. The patient, a 19-year-old girl with the characteristic mucocutaneous pigmentation of the Peutz–Jeghers syndrome, presented with abdominal pain. A large number of polyps were seen in the duodenum at endoscopy. Many of the larger polyps were removed with an endoscope which was manipulated into the jejunum at laparotomy

7.39 Carcinoid tumour A round filling defect is seen in the distal ileum. The 55-year-old man gave a one-year history of flushing and was found to have the carcinoid syndrome. Extensive investigations at another hospital including a barium follow-through examination were negative. The presence of a solitary primary carcinoid tumour in the distal ileum was confirmed at operation and metastases were present in the liver

7.40 Carcinoid tumour A large round intraluminal filling defect, with thickening of adjacent mucosal folds, is seen in the terminal ileum. The 66-year-old man presented with abdominal pain and on examination was found to have a small mass in the right iliac fossa. The presence of a mass in the distal ileum was confirmed at operation and on examination of the resected specimen proved to be a carcinoid tumour. No metastases were found at operation

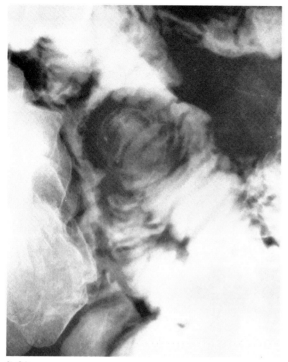

7.39

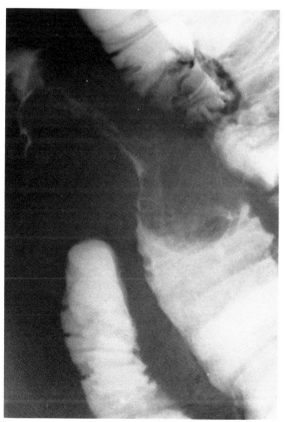

7.40

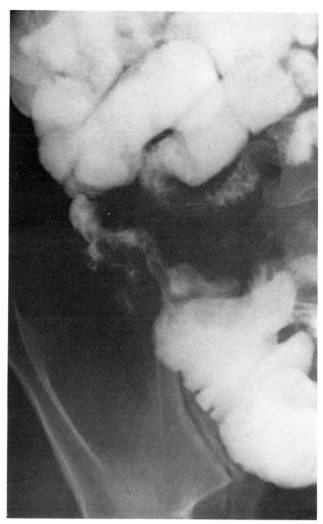

7.41

7.41 **Carcinoid tumour** There is a large infiltrating lesion in the distal ileum causing destruction of the normal mucosal pattern, marked irregular narrowing of the lumen and delay in the passage of barium. The 37-year-old man gave a four-year history of flushing provoked usually by alcohol. There was also marked hepatic enlargement and evidence of multiple metastatic deposits on a radionuclide scan

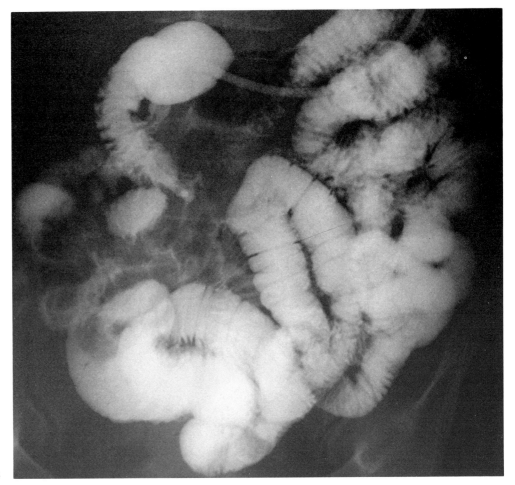

7.42a

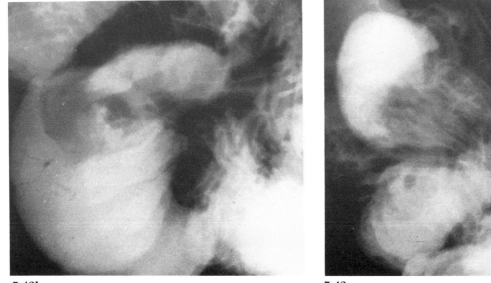

7.42b

7.42c

7.42 **Carcinoid tumour** a Compression, distortion and obstruction of the ileum is seen due to extensive infiltration and fibrosis by carcinoid tumour. b A *spot view* shows dilatation of a segment of ileum proximal to the infiltrated segment. c Thickened wall and thickened folds with sharp angulation are seen on this view. The patient, a 57-year-old man with a history of previous resection of ileum for carcinoid tumour, presented with the carcinoid syndrome, abdominal pain and diarrhoea

7.43 **Ileal lymphoma causing obstruction** a The jejunum and proximal ileum are distended and a narrowed distorted segment can be seen in the distal ileum. b A *spot view* shows the short narrowed segment with loss of mucosal pattern, shouldering of the margins and a large central ulcer crater. The patient, a 37-year-old woman with a 13-year history of follicular lymphoma, presented following two episodes of abdominal pain and vomiting. Plain abdominal radiographs showed no abnormality. The presence of an ulcerating follicular lymphoma of the ileum was confirmed on examination of the resected specimen.

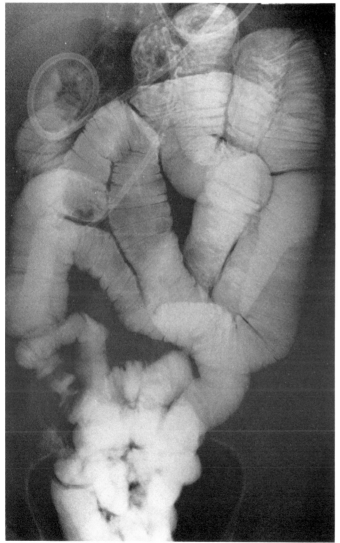

7.43a

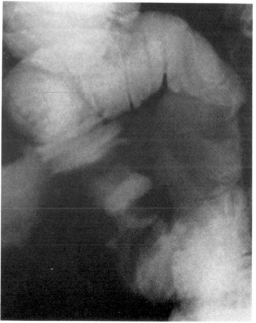

7.43b

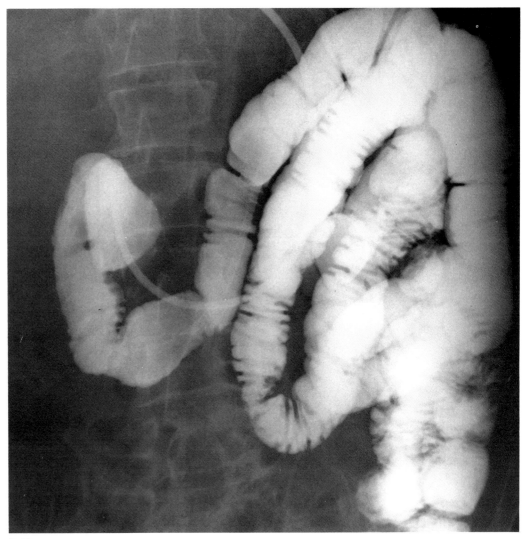

7.44a

7.44 **Lymphoma and coeliac disease** a The jejunum shows changes typical of coeliac disease with fewer and thinner valvulae conniventes than normal. b A long irregular infiltrating lesion is shown on this *spot view* of the ileum. The 64-year-old man presented with malabsorption six months before; coeliac disease was diagnosed on a jejunal biopsy. On this occasion he presented with symptoms suggesting intestinal obstruction. The ileal tumour proved to be a lymphosarcoma

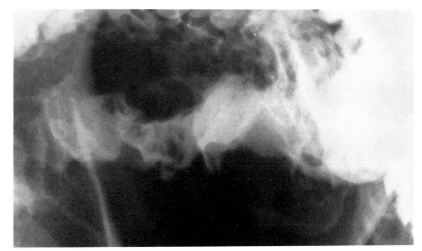

7.44b

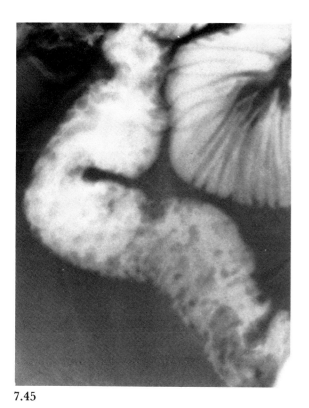

7.45

7.45 **Nodular lymphoid hyperplasia** Multiple, small round well-defined filling defects are seen in the terminal ileum of a 22-year-old female. Subsequent follow-up over three years yielded no evidence of organic disease

7.46 **Multiple lymphomatous deposits** *Spot views* of jejunum show a an irregular sessile polypoid filling defect, b two adjacent concentric infiltrating defects. The patient presented a month earlier as an emergency with free perforation. An ulcerating lesion that proved to be a lymphosarcoma was found at operation

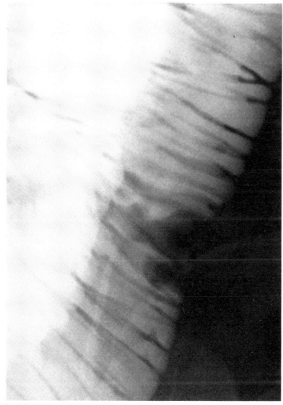

7.46a

7.46b

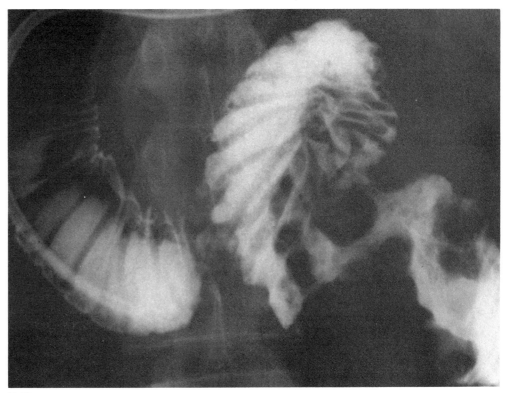

7.47

7.47 **Carcinoma** A large
irregular infiltrating lesion is
seen involving the proximal
jejunum. The 39-year- old man
presented with anaemia. At
operation a large tumour was
resected which proved to be a
carcinoma

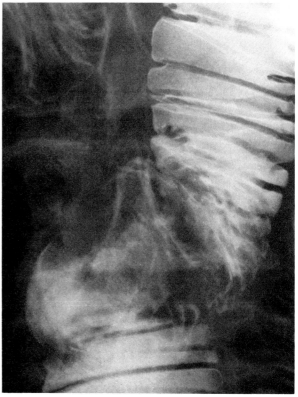

7.48

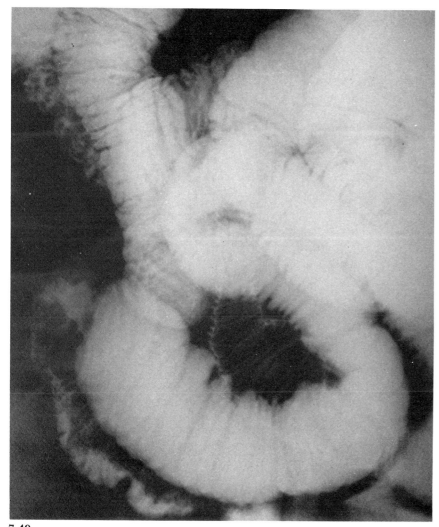

7.49

7.49 **Infiltrating carcinoma** An irregular infiltrating lesion is shown causing considerable narrowing of the lumen of a segment of ileum. Note the acute transition in calibre between the distended intestine proximally and the collapsed loops distal to the infiltrating lesion. There is also some dilatation of a short segment of intestine proximal to the lesion. The patient, a 56-year-old female with a history of previous resection for carcinoma of the colon, was admitted as an emergency with small intestinal obstruction. Two months before, a barium follow-through, performed because of similar symptoms, showed no abnormality. Infiltrating carcinoma involving the ileum was found at operation (Nolan & Marks 1981)

7.48 **Carcinoma** An irregular infiltrating lesion is seen on this view of a segment of jejunum; it proved to be a mixed adenosquamous carcinoma. The patient, a 59-year-old man with a history of adenomatous rectal polyps and a right hemicolectomy for carcinoma of the ascending colon, was admitted with melaena. At endoscopy a small polyp was seen in the duodenum which proved to be a tubular adenoma

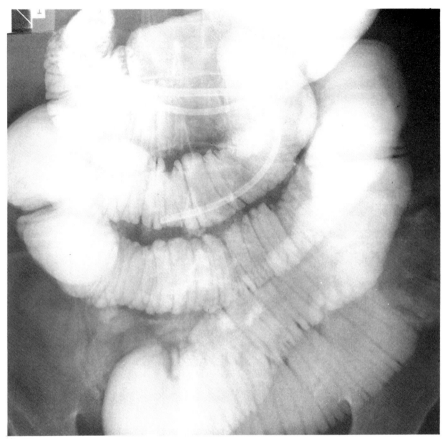

7.50a

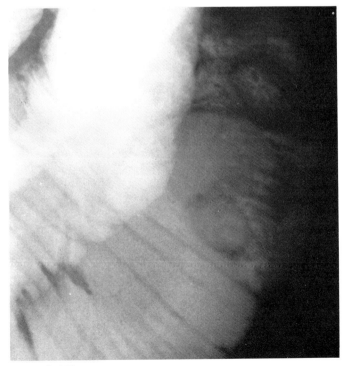

7.50b

7.50 **Infiltrating carcinoma causing obstruction** a The proximal jejunum is dilated and a mass is infiltrating a segment of jejunum on the left side. b A *spot view* of the obstructing lesion. The patient, a 74-year-old woman who had had a carcinoma of the colon resected two years before, was admitted with small intestinal obstruction. Infiltrating carcinoma of the colon involving the jejunum was found at operation

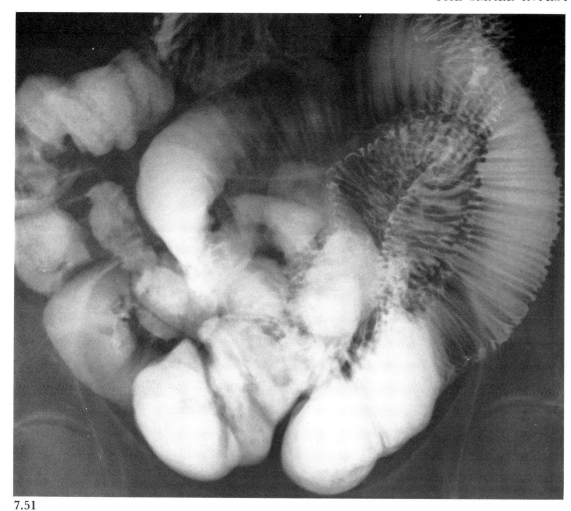

7.51

7.51 **Radiation enteritis** Extensive changes of radiation enteritis are seen involving the ileum. The pelvic loops of ileum are adherent to each other and there are multiple narrowed and distorted segments with loss of the normal mucosal pattern. Slight dilatation of the more proximal ileum due to partial obstruction is also seen. The valvulae conniventes of the slightly dilated segment are thickened and have the typical 'picket fence' outline. The patient, a 58-year-old female, had had a Wertheim's hysterectomy and radiation therapy for carcinoma of the uterus

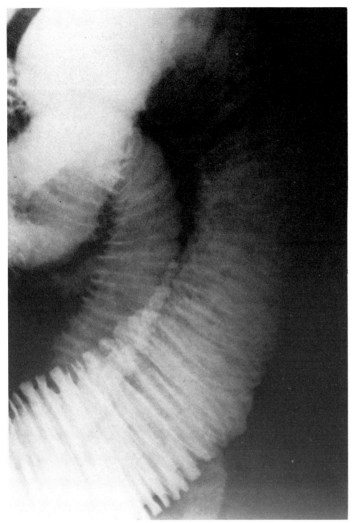

7.52

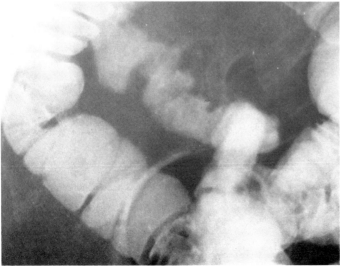

7.54

7.52 **Radiation enteritis** Barium outlines part of the jejunum and shows marked thickening of the valvulae conniventes in one loop. The more proximal segment is dilated due to obstruction. Similar changes were present throughout the small intestine. The patient, a 40-year-old woman, had had a Wertheim's hysterectomy and radiation therapy for carcinoma of both ovaries 13 years previously

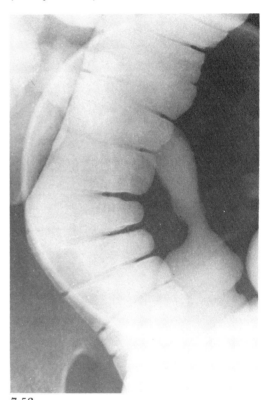

7.53

7.53 **Radiation stricture** This *spot view* shows a short narrowed segment in the distal ileum with dilatation of the more proximal ileum. No other changes of radiation enteritis were seen. The patient, a 69-year-old female who had had a Wertheim's hysterectomy with radium treatment for an extensive carcinoma of the cervix four years before, was admitted to hospital with symptoms of intestinal obstruction. Plain abdominal radiographs were normal. At operation there was no evidence of radiation damage in the remainder of the small intestine and the stricture was resected. Radiation damage localized to the site of the stricture was confirmed on histological examination. The patient made a complete recovery (Nolan & Marks 1981)

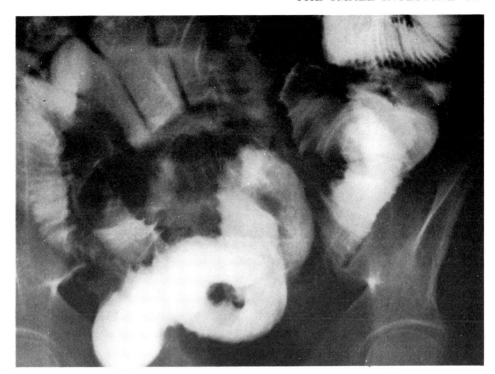

7.55a

7.55 **Acute ischaemia** a There is marked thickening of the mucosal folds throughout the ileum. b A *spot view* of a short segment. The 39-year-old female presented with acute abdominal pain six months after a right hemicolectomy for caecal volvulus. Her symptoms resolved rapidly and at a repeat examination three weeks later the small intestine had returned to normal

7.54 **Radiation stricture with ulceration** This *spot view* shows a short abnormal segment of ileum with loss of the normal mucosal pattern, narrowing and deformity. There was a slight delay in the passage of barium through the narrowed segment. The remainder of the small intestine was normal. Seven years earlier the patient had had a resection of an ovary and radiotherapy for carcinoma. This barium examination was carried out during the patient's fourth admission to hospital for suspected small intestinal obstruction. The plain abdominal radiographs were normal. At operation a short localized stricture with ulceration due to radiation damage was confirmed. A resection was performed and the patient made an uneventful recovery

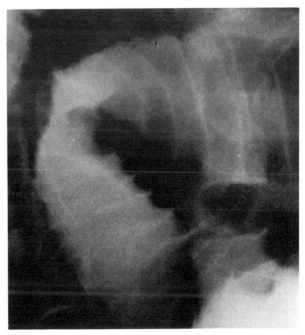

7.55b

7.56 **Chronic ischaemia** There is gross thickening of the valvulae conniventes and narrowing of the lumen in a segment of ileum. The patient, a 76-year-old female, presented with abdominal pain, flatulence and vomiting. At operation a mass of carcinoid tumour was found infiltrating the root of the mesentery and causing ischaemia

7.57 **Ischaemic stricture with perforation** There was considerable delay in the passage of barium through the distal jejunum and proximal ileum. Excess gas and fluid are seen in a dilated segment of ileum proximal to complete obstruction in a loop of ileum in the midline. A small leak of barium can be identified. The 30-year-old man was involved in a road traffic accident six weeks earlier and sustained multiple injuries. At operation a stricture with a localized perforation was seen at the site of a mesenteric tear. Histological examination of the resected specimen showed ischaemic necrosis of the wall of the intestine (Nolan & Marks 1981)

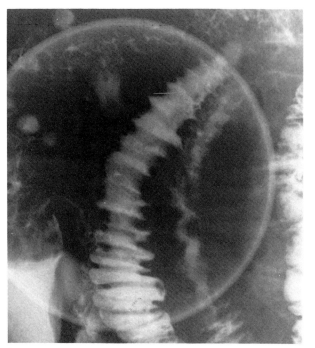

7.56

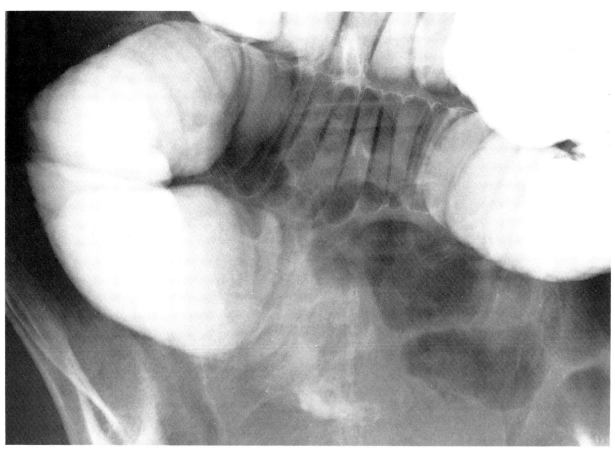

7.57

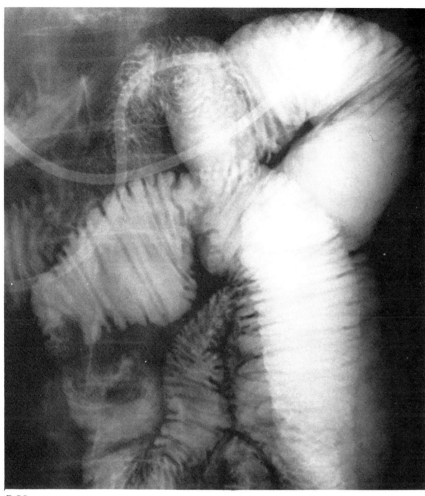

7.58a

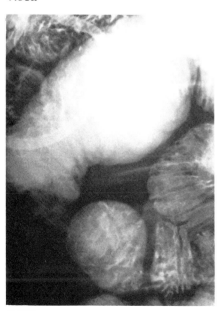

7.58b

7.58 Ischaemic stricture due to trauma a,b A short stricture of the jejunum is causing obstruction. There is an abrupt transition in calibre between the slightly dilated jejunum proximal to the stricture and the collapsed loops distally. The 33-year-old man had been admitted to hospital three months before with abdominal pain after being crushed against a wall for a few moments by the handle of a heavy roller. He was discharged within 24 hours. This examination was performed when he developed anorexia, abdominal pain, vomiting and weight loss. Histological examination of the resected specimen showed ischaemic damage of the circular muscle coat, with contraction and fibrosis

7.59 **Stricture caused by enteric-coated potassium tablets** A *retrograde barium examination* shows a short stricture (arrow) of the distal ileum. The patient presented with crampy abdominal pain. Plain abdominal radiographs and a barium follow-through showed no abnormality (Miller 1969)

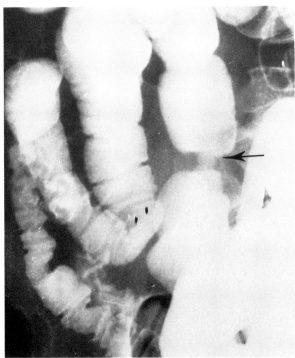

7.59

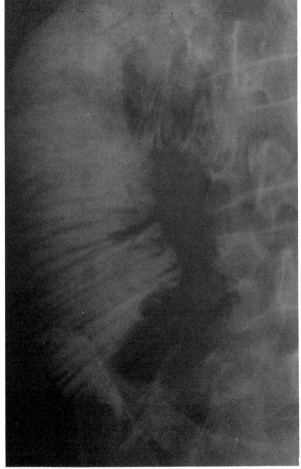

7.61

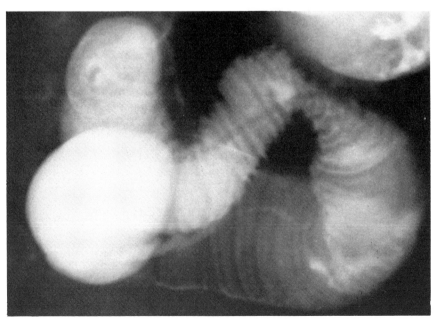

7.60

7.60 **Ischaemic stricture** A long markedly narrowed segment with proximal dilatation is seen in the proximal jejunum of a four-month-old baby that presented with vomiting and no previous history of illness. The pathologist considered the stricture was consistent with a healed ischaemic lesion, probably due to an episode of necrotizing enterocolitis. (Courtesy of Dr. Peter Stamper)

7.61 **Intramural haematoma** Large concentric filling defects a seen in the small intestine, causi obstruction in a patient on anticoagulant therapy (Courtesy Dr. W.J. Norman)

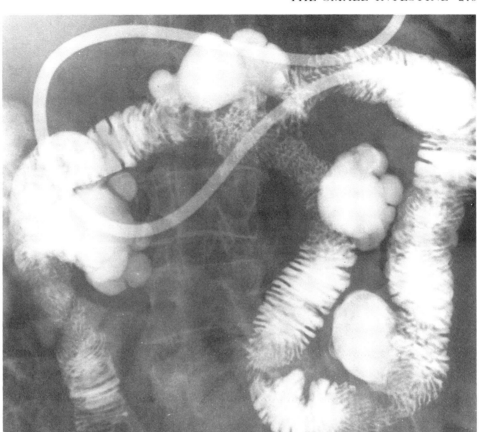

7.62a

7.62 Jejunal diverticula
a Multiple diverticula, some of
them multilobed, are shown in the
proximal jejunum. b A *spot view* of
one of the diverticula. The patient,
a 75-year-old female, was
investigated because of abdominal
pain

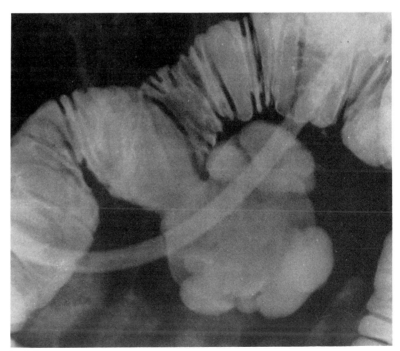

7.62b

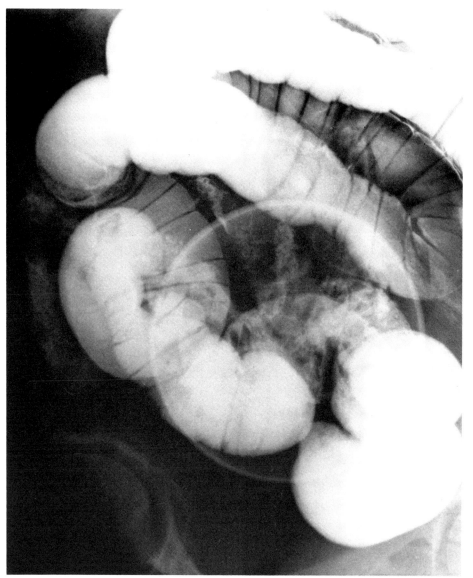

7.65

7.65 **Adhesions causing obstruction** There was considerable delay in the passage of barium. This *spot view* shows a sharp transition from dilated to collapsed loops of ileum in the right iliac fossa. The patient, a 29-year-old man who a year before had had an appendicectomy, presented with intestinal obstruction. Adhesions causing obstruction were found at operation

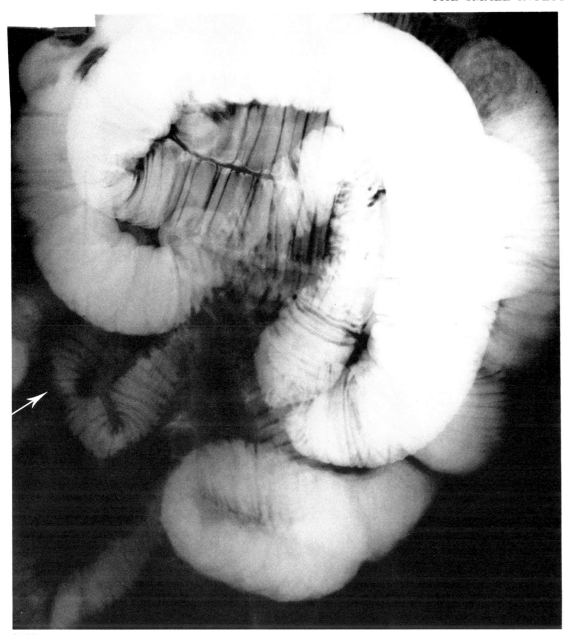

7.66

7.66 Adhesions causing obstruction Adhesions developed between a tube draining an appendix abscess (arrow) in the right iliac fossa and an adjacent loop of ileum. There is distension of the intestine proximal to the site of the adhesions and dilution of the barium by the intestinal fluid in the segment just proximal to the site of obstruction. The adhesions separated during the examination resulting in immediate relief of the obstruction (Nolan & Marks 1981)

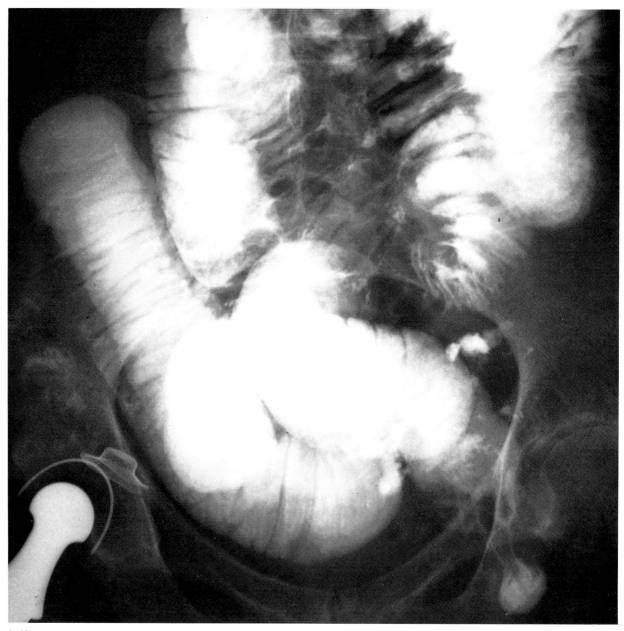

7.67

7.67 **Femoral hernia causing obstruction** A short
loop of small intestine is trapped in a left femoral hernia.
Dilatation of the intestine and dilution of the barium by
excess fluid are seen proximal to the site of obstruction.
This elderly female presented with obstruction two weeks
after a hip replacement; the hernia was not detected on
clinical examination (Nolan & Marks 1981)

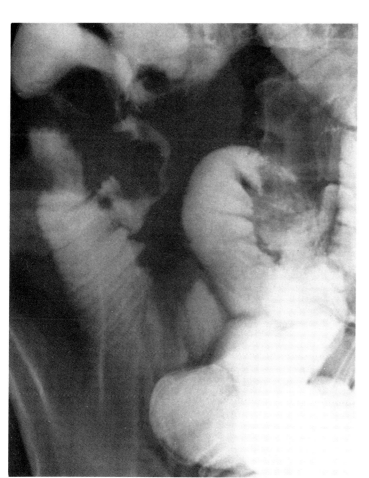

7.68

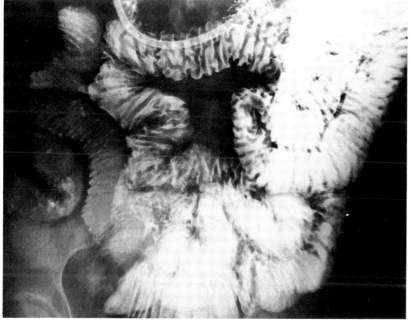

7.69

7.68 **Hernia through the lateral space around an ileostomy** A distorted, narrowed segment is seen just proximal to the ileostomy in a 34-year-old female who previously had a proctocolectomy for ulcerative colitis. The small intestine proximal to the site of obstruction is well-distended and contains excess fluid. The patient gave a two-year history of symptoms suggesting intermittent small intestinal obstruction. Two follow-through examinations, performed elsewhere, showed no abnormality. At operation a segment of ileum was found to have herniated through the lateral space adjacent to an ileostomy (Nolan & Marks 1981)

7.69 **Intestinal lymphangiectasia** Thickened valvulae conniventes are seen throughout most of the small intestine. The 21-year-old man with multiple haemangiomata, a mild left hemiparesis, hypertelorism and short stature developed malabsorption and steatorrhoea. Jejunal biopsy showed the typical changes of intestinal lymphangiectasia. (Courtesy of Dr. D.J. Lintott)

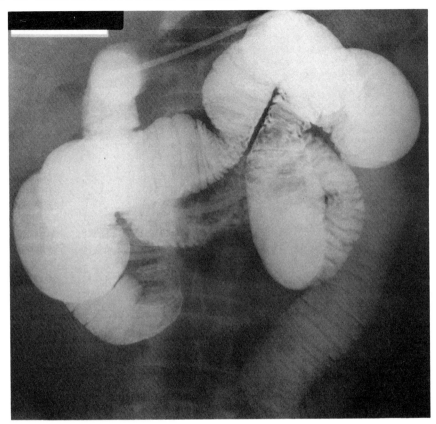

7.70a

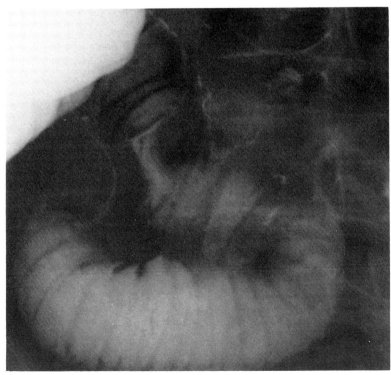

7.70b

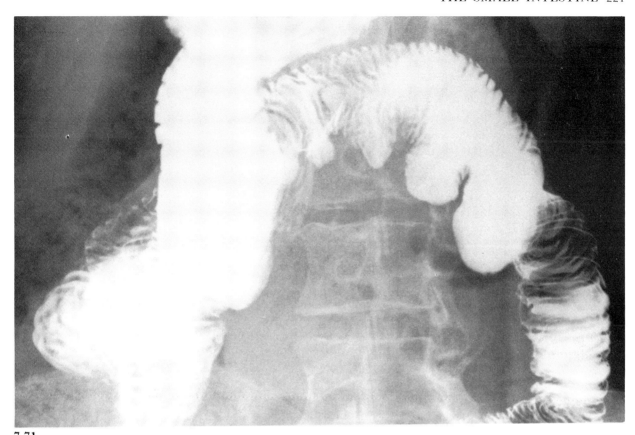

7.71

7.71 **Progressive systemic sclerosis** Localized dilatations are seen involving a segment of proximal jejunum in a patient with established progressive systemic sclerosis. (Courtesy of Dr. Myles McNulty)

7.70 **Band causing obstruction** a The jejunum is dilated and contains a large amount of fluid. Barium passed slowly through the small intestine. b A film taken 16 hours after the barium was infused shows marked narrowing of two adjacent short segments of ileum with a barium-filled loop in between. The patient, a 55-year-old man with no history of previous abdominal surgery was admitted with small intestinal obstruction. At operation a loop of ileum was found to be trapped by a band

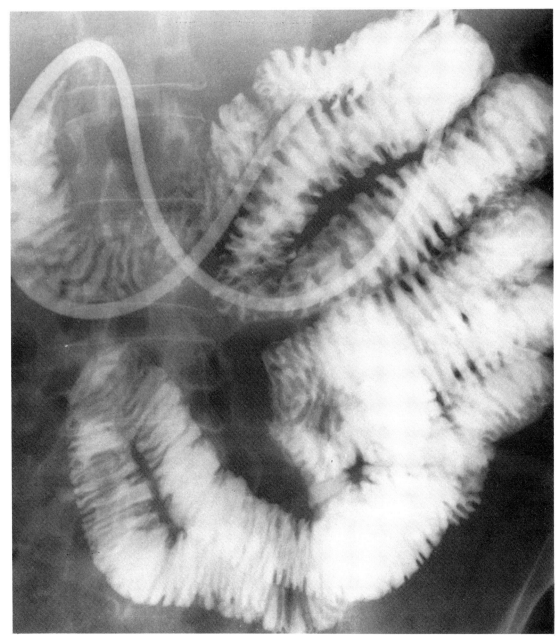

7.72

7.72 **Cirrhosis with mucosal oedema** There is thickening of the valvulae conniventes in the proximal jejunum in a patient with cirrhosis and portal hypertension

Tumours

Polyps Colonic polyps are mainly either tubular or villous adenomas. However, many are intermediate in structure and are classified as tubulovillous adenomas. Patients with adenomatous polyps usually present with rectal bleeding. Polyps are small, with a diameter of less than 2 cm, although they are occasionally larger. Radiologically they are seen as small, round, sessile or pedunculated filling defects in the colon. Multiple adenomatous polyps are often present.

Inflammatory polyps, often called pseudopolyps, are sometimes seen in the colon of patients with inflammatory bowel disease such as ulcerative colitis, Crohn's disease, amoebic colitis and schistosomiasis. They may be round or elongated and are often numerous. Inflammatory polyps may fuse together to form mucosal bridges.

Hyperplastic polyps are not uncommon in the colon; they are small, less than 0.5 cm in diameter, and are usually seen on the crest of a mucosal fold. They do not appear to have any malignant potential. Lipomas, hamartomas, neuromas and neurofibromas are other types of polyp infrequently present in the colon.

Intestinal polyposis syndromes The polyposis syndromes can be conveniently divided into hereditary and non-hereditary types (Table 8.1). Familial multiple polyposis, Gardner's polyposis and the Peutz–Jeghers syndrome are characterized by autosomal dominant inheritance (Dodds 1976). There is a strong family history of carcinoma in patients with familial polyposis. The polyps are not present at birth but develop during childhood or early adult life. Histologically they are of the adenomatous variety. Clinical features include rectal bleeding, diarrhoea and abdominal pain; carcinoma tends to have developed by the time symptoms present. Barium enema examination shows many polyps throughout the colon sometimes with an associated carcinoma. Patients with the condition will almost invariably develop carcinoma of the colon and prophylactic colectomy is indicated.

Gardner's syndrome is characterized by multiple soft tissue tumours, skeletal osteomas and polyposis coli. The adenomatous polyps are similar in every way to those seen in familial polyposis and patients develop carcinoma of the colon unless a prophylactic colectomy is performed.

Table 8.1   Intestinal polyposis syndromes (Dodds 1976)

A. Hereditary
   1. Familial multiple polyposis
   2. Gardner's syndrome
   3. Peutz–Jeghers syndrome
   4. Turcot's syndrome

B. Non-hereditary
   1. Cronkhite–Canada syndrome
   2. Juvenile polyposis (occasionally hereditary)

8 The Colon and Rectum

Combined mucocutaneous pigmentation and gastrointestinal polyposis are present in the Peutz–Jeghers syndrome. The abnormal pigmentation is pathognomonic. Brown or black, oval or slightly irregular macules, 1–5 mm in diameter, are characteristically present on the mucosal surface of the lower lip and on the buccal mucosa (Dodds 1976). Pigmentation may also occur on the face and the volar aspects of the hands and feet. Presenting symptoms include abdominal pain, intussusception and rectal bleeding. The small intestine is the usual site but the colon and stomach are involved in one-quarter of patients with the syndrome. The polyps in the small intestine are hamartomatous malformations with no malignant potential while the colonic polyps are adenomatous and carcinomas do occur.

Turcot's syndrome is a rare condition characterized by the association of central nervous tumours—nearly all supratentorial glioblastomas—and multiple adenomatous polyps of the colon (Turcot *et al.* 1959; Dodds 1976). It appears to have an autosomal recessive mode of inheritance.

Juvenile polyposis normally presents in childhood. The polyps are retention or inflammatory polyps and have characteristic gross and histological appearances (Dodds 1976). They have a smooth round contour, are often haemorrhagic and the cut surface reveals cystic spaces filled with mucin. Juvenile polyps are seen in children, mainly in the colon, but sometimes in the stomach or small intestine. The polyps are mostly solitary and rectal bleeding is the usual presenting feature. They have no malignant potential and have a tendency towards autoamputation or regression.

Cronkhite and Canada in 1955 described a syndrome of generalized gastrointestinal polyposis, alopecia, pigmentation and atrophy of the finger and toe nails. The characteristic features develop in middle or old age when patients present with anorexia, abdominal pain, weight loss and watery diarrhoea, sometimes containing blood. Polyps are present in the stomach, small intestine and colon. They show inflammatory changes of the juvenile type and have no malignant potential. Spontaneous remission can occur but most patients become weak as a result of electrolyte and calcium loss, develop hypoproteinaemia and die within 18 months of the onset of symptoms.

Carcinoma Colorectal carcinoma is one of the most common forms of malignant disease and is. second only to lung cancer as a cause of death in England and Wales. The incidence is high in populations with good socioeconomic standards where diet appears to play an important role, and low in poorer areas of the world. Obstructive symptoms, rectal bleeding, iron deficiency anaemia and change in bowel habit are the most common presenting features.

Plain abdominal radiographs should be the initial investigation for patients who present with symptoms or signs of intestinal obstruction. The barium examination of the colon is the most important diagnostic procedure and when properly performed is accurate at detecting primary cancers of the colon that are beyond the reach of the sigmoidoscope. The double-contrast barium enema should be used routinely for this purpose. Radionuclide studies, ultrasound and computerized tomography are used for detecting the presence of hepatic metastases.

Early diagnosis is of the utmost importance as the survival rate is much higher if the condition is detected at an early stage. When the carcinoma has spread into the tissues of the bowel wall, but not beyond the muscularis propria and there are no lymph node metastases (Dukes 'A'), the patient is almost invariably cured of his disease by appropriate surgical treatment (Morson & Dawson 1979). If the growth has spread beyond the muscularis propria into the pericolic or perirectal tissues in continuity, but there are no regional lymph node metastases (Dukes 'B'), there is a 70 per cent chance of being cured. Once the lymph nodes are involved the prognosis is poor with only a one in three chance of the patient surviving five years. There is evidence that carcinomas of the colon arise from previously benign adenomas (Muto *et al.* 1975).

Radiologically there are two principal appearances of primary carcinoma of the colon—the infiltrating lesion which is the type most often seen, and the polypoid filling defect. Carcinomas are seen infiltrating and distorting part of the wall of the colon or rectum with destruction of the normal mucosal pattern. In more advanced cases the infiltrating carcinoma is an annular growth involving the complete circumference of the colon thus causing stenosis. The normal mucosal pattern of the narrowed segment is completely destroyed, the lumen is irregular and there is often shouldering of the upper and lower margins of the tumour. Polypoid carcinomas are large and irregular and often fill the lumen of the involved segment of colon.

It may be impossible to differentiate between benign polyps and polypoid carcinoma on the radiological appearances alone. Radiological features of polypoid lesions that suggest malignancy include dimpling or indentation at the base, and an irregular surface

(Welin & Welin 1976). If the width at the base of the polyp is greater than the height and the outline of the polyp *en face* is oval the growth is more likely to be malignant. Five per cent of patients with carcinoma of the colon or rectum will have more than one primary carcinoma at the time of diagnosis (Morson & Dawson 1979). Adenomatous polyps are frequently present in the colon of patients with carcinoma. Multiple tumours, adenomas or adenocarcinomas were present synchronously in 20 per cent of patients in one survey (Muto *et al.* 1975).

Patients with familial polyposis coli have a high incidence of carcinoma of the colon and there is also an increased incidence in patients with ulcerative colitis. The carcinomas in ulcerative colitis are often multiple and arise predominantly on the left side of the colon and there is a higher incidence of high-grade and colloid carcinomas.

Lymphoma The colon and rectum are occasionally the site of lymphomatous tumours.

Metastatic tumour The colon can be infiltrated by metastatic tumour. Intraperitoneal spread preferentially affects the pouch of Douglas, the sigmoid colon and the ileocaecal region (Meyers 1973). Direct extension can occur from neighbouring organs or along structures such as lymph channels (Lammer *et al.* 1981). Haematogenous spread along the mesenteric attachment can occur (Meyers 1973). Metastatic involvement of the colon may give appearances similar to inflammatory bowel disease, particularly Crohn's disease.

Diverticular disease

Colonic diverticula are false diverticula that result from herniation of the mucosa and submucosa through the circular muscle layer. The sigmoid colon is the site most frequently involved and they often involve the descending colon. Until recently diverticula of the right half of the colon were an uncommon finding but nowadays barium enema examinations frequently show diverticula of the ascending and the transverse colon.

In most cases diverticula are asymptomatic although diverticular disease may give rise to diarrhoea or change in bowel habit. Bleeding with acute haemorrhage is a well-recognized complication. Diverticular disease is the most frequent cause of acute rectal bleeding and angiography is the best investigation for such patients. Inflammation with abscess formation is another complication of diverticular disease. It can lead to perforation, abscess or mass formation, or development of a sinus track or fistula to the bladder, vagina, small intestine or skin.

Great care is required when performing a barium enema on patients with a suspected diverticular abscess; only a small amount of barium should be used and at low pressure. Radiologically diverticula are seen on barium enema studies as small out-pouchings of the colon when viewed in profile. The *en face* view shows them as small collections of barium with a sharp outer and a poorly defined inner margin, unlike polyps which have a sharp inner and a poorly defined outer margin.

Diverticular masses secondary to abscess formation may compress the wall of the intestine causing obstruction. Features which help differentiate a diverticular mass from carcinoma of the colon are an absence of shouldering of the margins and the presence of normal mucosa in the narrowed segment. Recognizing multiple colonic diverticula in patients with a mass is of little help as carcinoma and diverticula frequently coexist. Small carcinomas and polyps may be difficult to detect at barium enema examination if a large number of diverticula are present causing overlapping shadows. Colonoscopy is indicated where the clinical symptoms suggest carcinoma or polyps but the double-contrast enema shows only severe diverticular disease.

Traction diverticula Traction diverticula of the caecum and ascending colon may be seen in association with calcified tuberculous mesenteric lymph nodes (Nolan *et al.* 1971). These diverticula are lobulated and larger than the usual colonic diverticula. The base is adjacent to a number of calcified lymph glands and mucosal folds can be clearly seen passing into the diverticula.

Inflammatory bowel disease

Ulcerative colitis Ulcerative colitis is a condition of unknown aetiology characterized by diffuse inflammation of part or all of the wall of the rectum and colon (Truelove & Reynell 1972). The disease may be limited to the rectum or it may involve the rectum and a varying length of proximal colon in continuity. Sometimes the whole colon is involved. The disease usually pursues an intermittent or chronic course.

The majority of patients develop the disease in early adult life presenting with diarrhoea and blood in the motions. Varying degrees of constitutional disturbance accompany the colonic symptoms depending on the severity and extent of the inflammation. The complications of an acute attack are massive haemorrhage, perforation and toxic megacolon. The most significant late complication is the development of carcinoma of the colon. Features of ulcerative colitis which are associated with a high risk of developing carcinoma include a clinically severe first attack, involvement of the whole colon and continuous chronic symptoms (Edwards & Truelove 1964). Patients prone to develop carcinoma are those in whom the colitis developed in youth or in whom ulcerative colitis has been present for more than 20 years. Stricture formation is uncommon in ulcerative colitis but it can occur as a late complication.

Plain abdominal radiographs are particularly helpful in the investigation of an acute attack (Bartram 1976). If intracolonic air is present the mucosal state can be accurately assessed, especially in toxic megacolon where the mucosal islands are well demonstrated on plain abdominal radiographs. A modified barium enema can be performed to assess acute colitis. Preparation is not required as faecal residue does not accumulate adjacent to an actively inflamed mucosa. The use of catheters with an inflatable balloon is contraindicated in the presence of active inflammatory disease of the colon (Thomas 1979). Barium is infused carefully into the rectum under low pressure until the head of the column reaches the caecum or begins to outline a segment containing faeces. If there is evidence of severe mucosal ulceration, radiographs of the inflamed segment are obtained. In patients where the mucosa is not severely inflamed barium is drained off, air is introduced and double-contrast radiographs are obtained.

To assess the colon in patients with chronic ulcerative colitis a double-contrast enema is performed following adequate preparation. The appearances on the barium enema will depend on the extent and severity of the disease. Patients with mild colitis have the normal smooth mucosal pattern replaced by a slightly granular pattern; patients with inflammation of moderate severity show moderate mucosal ulceration. In severe cases the ulceration is marked and may be undermining the mucosa. The haustral pattern of the colon is usually absent in moderate or severe colitis. A smooth featureless outline, shortening of the colon and narrowing of the lumen are signs seen in chronic ulcerative colitis. Inflammatory polyps may also be present or there may be evidence of active disease.

Crohn's disease of the colon The radiological signs of Crohn's disease in the colon are the same as those seen in the small intestine (Chapter 7). There is often predominant involvement of the right half of the colon with the disease. Discrete ulcers in the colon are shown as small collections of barium with surrounding zones of translucency due to oedema.

The mucosa between the discrete ulcers is normal, which helps distinguish Crohn's colitis from ulcerative colitis. In ulcerative colitis the whole mucosa shows a granular pattern due to ulceration. Fissure ulcers, longitudinal ulcers and cobblestoning are seen in Crohn's disease. The most common site of sinus and fistula formation is the anal region. Stenosis, asymmetrical involvement, skip lesions and inflammatory polyps occur. Evidence of Crohn's disease involving the terminal ileum or indentation of the medial wall of the caecum by the thickened wall of the terminal ileum or by swollen lymph glands may be seen on the barium enema.

An appearance that has received little attention but may represent one of the early signs of Crohn's disease is the transverse stripes described by Welin and Welin (1976). The stripe effect is caused by contrast medium lodging in deep furrows between swollen mucosal folds and is seen on double-contrast barium studies as transverse straight lines of barium. The stripes are not a feature of ulcerative colitis and can be useful for differentiating Crohn's disease from ulcerative colitis.

Tuberculosis The radiological appearances of ileocaecal tuberculosis are discussed in the previous chapter. Tuberculosis may involve the caecal pole and be shown on barium enema examination as a circumferential filling defect. Distal to the ileocaecal area tuberculosis may cause colonic strictures; in some cases the strictures are multiple (Chawla et al. 1971).

Amoebiasis Amoebiasis is common in the tropics but there are numerous cases on record in patients who have never left the United Kingdom (Cook 1980). Acute or intermittent diarrhoea, with blood and mucus, is the usual initial symptom, sometimes accompanied by headache, nausea, chills, fever and colic. Fulminating invasive amoebiasis of the colon may cause toxic megacolon, perforation or stricture formation (Cardoso et al. 1977). In less severe cases the barium enema shows segments of small ulcers and nodules. The lesions are patchy with areas of adjacent intact mucosa (Cockshott & Middlemiss 1979). The caecum, ascending colon, sigmoid colon and rectum are the parts most frequently involved. Amoebomas are seen as irregular, segmental filling defects that may be multiple.

Schistosomiasis The colon may show changes in patients infected with schistosomiasis, particularly Schistosoma mansoni. Polyps, 1–2 cm in diameter, in the sigmoid colon and rectum are the most frequent finding, although the descending and transverse colon may be involved (Cockshott & Middlemiss 1979). Mucosal ulcers and areas or segments of narrowing may also be seen.

Lymphogranuloma venerium Intestinal lymphogranuloma is a common condition in the West Indies. There are two stages of the disease (Annamunthodo & Marryatt 1961), one of which is proctocolitis where the main symptoms are those of colitis and the appearances on barium enema show loss of the haustral pattern. The changes usually affect the whole colon, often unevenly. The other stage of the disease is when an anorectal stricture and marked shortening develop involving the rectum and a varying length of sigmoid colon. Perianal sinuses, fistulae and abscesses often complicate the stenotic stage. Fistulae between the anorectal region and the lower vagina are frequently present.

Pseudomembranous enterocolitis Pseudomembranous enterocolitis is an inflammatory condition of the large intestine, sometimes involving the small intestine, which is characterized by the formation of a membrane of mucus, fibrin and inflammatory cells adherent to the mucosal surface. It often follows the use of broad-spectrum antibiotics such as lincomycin and clindamycin (Scott *et al.* 1973). The condition is believed to result from an overgrowth of a cytotoxic strain of *Clostridium difficile*. The usual presenting feature is an acute onset of diarrhoea, often with blood and excessive amounts of mucus. Patients may become severely ill with the condition. Pseudomembranous enterocolitis should always be considered in the differential diagnosis of ulcerative colitis.

The diagnosis is made by sigmoidoscopy and biopsy combined with radiological studies. Apart from inflammation, whitish plaques of mucous membrane are seen. The essential pathological feature appears to be mucosal ischaemia of the intestine caused by fibrin plugging of the capillaries (Whitehead 1971). Plain radiographs may show gas-filled loops of small and large intestine with thickening of the haustrations of the colon (Cohen *et al.* 1974). There may be evidence of severe spasm on barium enema examination. The margin is often serrated with multiple irregular defects; thickening of the haustra and a nodular pattern due to oedema may be seen (Nolan *et al.* 1976).

Ischaemic colitis The main clinical features of ischaemic colitis are the sudden onset of abdominal pain, rectal bleeding and signs of left-sided peritonitis (Marston *et al.* 1966). The characteristic radiological signs are narrowing and marked mucosal oedema giving a classical 'thumb-printing' appearance. Usually a single segment of splenic flexure with adjacent transverse and descending colon is involved. The affected large intestine either returns to normal or a stricture develops.

Neonatal necrotizing enterocolitis This is a condition that occurs primarily in premature or low-birth-weight infants, characterized clinically by abdominal distension, vomiting, absent bowel sounds and blood in the stools (Virjee *et al.* 1979). The findings on plain abdominal radiographs include separation of bowel loops (mucosal oedema, haemorrhage or free intraperitoneal fluid), intramural gas, dilated bowel loops, free intraperitoneal gas or portal vein gas. Stricture formation as a late complication may be seen in up to 25 per cent of cases of necrotizing enterocolitis. Strictures may be multiple particularly in the colon.

Behcet's colitis Colitis occurs occasionally in Behcet's syndrome. Controversy exists as to whether these cases represent true involvement of the colon by Behcet's disease, are coincidental inflammatory bowel disease or whether Behcet's syndrome is an autoimmune phenomenon associated with inflammatory bowel disease (Smith *et al.* 1973).

Other conditions

Radiation injury to the colon The distal sigmoid colon and rectum is the most frequent site of radiation damage to the large intestine. Patients present with rectal bleeding or obstruction. Elongated narrowing of the rectum and sigmoid colon is the most common radiological manifestation on barium enema examination (Rogers & Goldstein 1977). In some cases fistulae to adjacent organs may be present.

Endometriosis The serosal surface of the colon and terminal ileum may be the site of endometrial deposits (Theander & Wehlin 1961). Deformity and narrowing, particularly of the lower sigmoid colon, may be seen on the barium enema. The changes often persist after the menopause.

Idiopathic megacolon Idiopathic megacolon is the term applied to severe constipation developing in childhood in the absence of organic disease (Lumsden & Truelove 1965). It may be difficult to differentiate from Hirschsprung's disease. The colon may become considerably distended and persist so into adult life. Sigmoid volvulus is a frequent complication of idiopathic megacolon.

Pneumatosis coli Pneumatosis intestinalis, a condition characterized by the presence of gas cysts in the wall of the intestine, can involve any part of the gastrointestinal tract but the colon is the most common site (Gruenberg *et al.* 1979). The condition may be associated with chronic obstructive airway disease. Patients often present with diarrhoea and the diagnosis is made on sigmoidoscopy or barium enema examination. The sigmoid colon and the descending colon are most frequently involved. In some cases the diagnosis can be made on plain abdominal radiographs when grape-like radiolucent clusters are seen along the contour of the colon and in the region of the mesentery (Marshak *et al.* 1977). Barium enema examination shows multiple small gas-filled cysts indenting the wall of the colon.

Progressive systemic sclerosis There are characteristic changes in the colon of about one-half of patients with progressive systemic sclerosis (scleroderma). The changes include pseudodiverticula which are seen best in the transverse and descending colon, areas of rigidity between the sacculations, and in advanced cases the pseudodiverticula disappear and are replaced by a dilated and atonic colon (Kemp Harper & Jackson 1965).

Irritable colon Irritable colon is a common functional disturbance attributable to spasm. Abdominal pain and diarrhoea are the clinical presenting features. Barium studies are undertaken to exclude any organic cause for the patient's symptoms.

Cathartic colon The prolonged and excessive use of irritant cathartics can cause characteristic radiological changes in the distal ileum and colon (Jewell & Kline 1954). The terminal ileum becomes dilated and the ileocaecal valve is wide open. The right side of the colon is more markedly involved and is shown to be atonic with loss of the haustral pattern and almost complete absence of the hepatic flexure. Segments of persistent contraction may be seen. The left side of the colon may be normal in appearance.

Appendicitis Radiology can be of value in some cases of acute appendicitis. Plain radiographs may show thickening of the wall of the caecum, dilatation of the caecum or a fluid level in the caecum. Fluid levels may also be present in the terminal ileum. The combination of caecal and terminal ileal dilatation with fluid levels and haziness due to free fluid—appendiceal ileus—is highly suggestive of acute appendicitis (Soter 1973). The appendix is likely to be gangrenous or perforated if appendix calculi are seen in the presence of clinical symptoms of appendicitis. Occasionally gas is seen in the lumen of the appendix in acute gangrenous appendicitis. Supporting signs include loss of the right psoas shadow, loss of the properitoneal fat line, free air in the peritoneal cavity and signs of small bowel ileus.

The barium enema examination can be very helpful in patients with suspected acute appendicitis when the clinical signs and plain radiographs are not diagnostic (Soter 1973). Preparation is not required and the barium is infused under low pressure. If there is filling and visualization of the complete length of the appendix, acute appendicitis can be excluded. Non-filling of the lumen of the appendix is not diagnostic unless there are associated changes of the caecum and terminal ileum. A sharp irregular cut-off of the barium in the appendix shows definite evidence of obstruction of part of the appendix lumen. There may be indentation of the caecum, or extrinsic pressure on the lateral aspect of the terminal ileum. An inverted appendix stump may be seen at barium enema examination in patients who have had a previous appendicectomy.

Mucocele of the appendix Mucocele of the appendix occurs when there is obstruction of the appendix lumen and mucus continues to be produced behind the obstruction. Patients present with right lower quadrant discomfort. On examination a mass may be palpable. Calcification in the wall or lumen of a cyst may occasionally be seen on plain abdominal radiographs. A round, well-defined filling defect in the caecum with non-visualization of the appendix are the characteristic features on barium enema examination (Watne & Trevino 1962; Nolan 1977).

References

Annamunthodo H. & Marryatt J. (1961) Barium studies in intestinal lymphogranuloma venerium. *Br. J. Radiol.*, **34**, 53

Bartram C.I. (1976) Plain abdominal X-ray in acute colitis. *J. R. Soc. Med.*, **69**, 617

Cardoso J.M., Kimura K., Stoopen M., Cervantes L.F., Elizondo L., Churchill R. & Moncada R. (1977) Radiology of invasive amoebiasis of the colon. *Am. J. Roentgenol.*, **128**, 935

Chawla S., Mukerjee P. & Bery K. (1971) Segmental tuberculosis of the colon. *Clin. Radiol.*, **22**, 104

Cockshott P. & Middlemiss H. (1979) *Clinical Radiology in the Tropics*. Edinburgh: Churchill Livingstone

Cohen L.E., Smith C.J., Pister J.D. & Wells R.F. (1974) Clindamycin (Cleocin) colitis. *Am. J. Roentgenol.*, **121**, 301

Cook G.C. (1980) *Tropical Gastroenterology*. Oxford: Oxford University Press

Cronkhite L.W. Jr. & Canada W.J. (1955) Generalized gastrointestinal polyposis: an unusual syndrome of polyposis, pigmentation, alopecia and onychotrophia. *N. Engl. J. Med.*, **252**, 1011

Dodds W.J. (1976) Clinical and roentgen features of the intestinal polyposis syndromes. *Gastrointest. Radiol.*, **1**, 127

Edwards F.C. & Truelove S.C. (1964) The course and prognosis of ulcerative colitis. *Gut*, **5**, 1

Gruenberg J.C., Grodinsky C. & Ponka J.L. (1979) Pneumatosis intestinalis. *Dis. Colon Rectum*, **22**, 5

Jewell F.C. & Kline J.R. (1954) The purged colon. *Radiology*, **62**, 368

Kemp Harper R.A. & Jackson D.C. (1965) Progressive systemic sclerosis. *Br. J. Radiol.*, **38**, 825

Lammer J., Dirschmid K. & Hügel H. (1981) Carcinomatous metastases to the colon simulating Crohn's disease. *Gastrointest. Radiol.*, **6**, 89

Lumsden K. & Truelove S.C. (1965) *Radiology of the Digestive System*. Oxford: Blackwell Scientific Publications

Marshak R.H., Lindner A.E. & Maklansky D. (1977) Pneumatosis cystoides coli. *Gastrointest. Radiol.*, **2**, 85

Marston A., Murray T.P., Lea Thomas M. & Morson B.C. (1966) Ischaemic colitis. *Gut*, **7**, 1

Meyers M.A. (1973) Distribution of intra-abdominal malignant seeding: dependency on dynamics of flow of ascitic fluid. *Am. J. Roentgenol.*, **119**, 198

Morson B.C. & Dawson I.M.P. (1979) *Gastrointestinal Pathology*, Oxford: Blackwell Scientific Publications

Muto T., Bussey H.J.R. & Morson B.C. (1975) The evolution of cancer of the colon and rectum. *Cancer*, **36**, 2251

Nolan D.J. (1977) Caecal mass. *J. Am. Med. Assoc.*, **237**, 371

Nolan D.J. (1982) *Radiological Assessment in Recent Results in Cancer Research*, Vol. 83, *Colorectal Cancer* (Ed. Duncan W.) Berlin: Springer Verlag

Nolan D.J., Goodman M.J. & Skinner J.M. (1976) Pseudomembranous enterocolitis. *J. R. Soc. Med.*, **69**, 621

Nolan D.J., Norman W.J. & Airth G.R. (1971) Traction diverticula of the colon. *Clin. Radiol.*, **22**, 458

Rogers L.F. & Goldstein H.M. (1977) Roentgen manifestations of radiation injury to the gastrointestinal tract. *Gastrointest. Radiol.*, **2**, 281

Scott A.J., Nicholson G.I. & Kerr A.R. (1973) Lincomycin as a cause of pseudomembranous colitis. *Lancet*, **ii**, 1232

Smith G.E., Kime L.R. & Pitcher J.L. (1973) The colitis of Behcet's disease: a separate entity? *Am. J. Dig. Dis.*, **18**, 987

Soter C.S. (1973) The contribution of the radiologist to the diagnosis of acute appendicitis. *Semin. Roentgenol.* **8**, 375

Theander G. & Wehlin L. (1961) Deformation of the recto-sigmoid junction in pelvic endometriosis. *Acta Radiol.*, **55**, 241

Thomas B.M. (1979) The instant enema in inflammatory bowel disease. *Clin. Radiol.*, **30**, 165

Truelove S.C. & Reynell P.C. (1972) *Diseases of the Digestive System*. Oxford: Blackwell Scientific Publications

Turcot J., Després J. & St. Pierre F. (1959) Malignant tumours of the nervous system associated with familial polyposis of the colon: report of two cases. *Dis. Colon Rectum*, **2**, 465

Virjee J., Somers S., DeSa D. & Stevenson G. (1979) Changing patterns of neonatal necrotizing enterocolitis. *Gastrointest. Radiol.*, **4**, 169

Watne A.L. & Trevino E. (1962) Diagnostic features of mucocele of the appendix. *Arch. Surg.*, **84**, 516

Welin S. & Welin G. (1976) *The Double-Contrast Examination of the Colon. Experience with the Welin Modification*. Stuttgart: George Thieme

Whitehead R. (1971) Ischaemic enterocolitis: an expression of the intravascular coagulation syndrome. *Gut*, **12**, 912

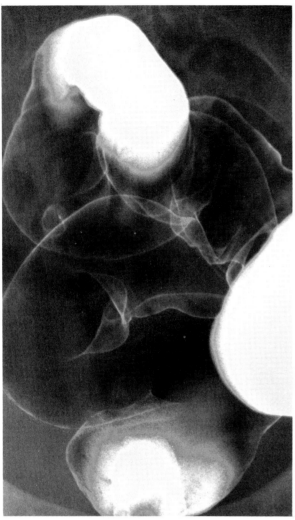

8.1

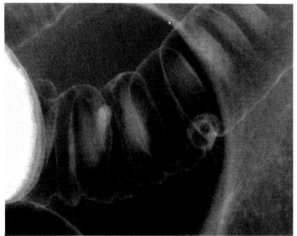

8.2

8.1 Adenomatous polyp in the distal sigmoid Note the clear inner margin of the barium surrounding the slightly irregular base of the polyp on double-contrast barium examination. The patient presented with a three-week history of diarrhoea and blood per rectum. The polyp was removed at endoscopy and proved to be a tubular adenoma

8.2 Adenomatous polyp A small polyp less than 1 cm in diameter is seen in the sigmoid colon. The patient gave a short history of passing blood per rectum. The polyp was removed at colonoscopy and proved to be a tubular adenoma

8.3 Pedunculated polyp A large polyp, over 2 cm in diameter, is seen at the rectosigmoid junction. The patient gave a one-year history of loose bowel motions. It was removed at sigmoidoscopy and reported as an adenomatous polyp

8.4 Adenomatous polyp of the caecum The patient, a 56-year-old female, gave a long history of ulcerative colitis. A *spot view* of the caecum taken during barium enema examination shows a moderate-sized, slightly irregular polypoid filling defect in the caecum which was reported as a carcinoma. A colectomy was performed and the polypoid lesion proved to be a villous adenoma with surrounding dysplasia

8.5 Benign adenomatous polyp A barium examination was performed because the patient gave a history of diarrhoea and abdominal pain. A moderate-sized, irregular polypoid lesion with a wide base is shown on the medial aspect of the descending limb of the splenic flexure. It was considered to be a carcinoma and a left hemicolectomy was performed. The lesion proved to be a tubulovillous adenoma with no evidence of malignancy

8.6 Pedunculated adenomatous polyp A large, slightly irregular polyp is seen on a pedicle in the hepatic flexure. The patient presented following an episode of acute rectal bleeding. The polyp was removed at endoscopy. On histological examination it proved to be a tubulovillous adenoma with substantial dysplasia and probable malignant degeneration within the polyp but no invasion of underlying tissue

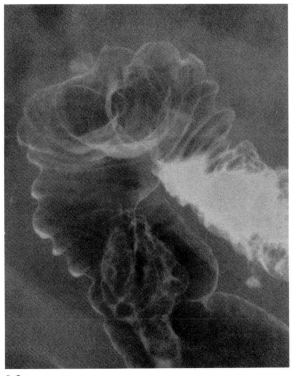

8.3

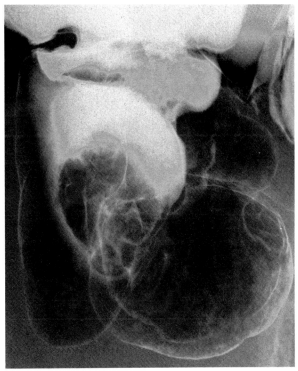

8.4

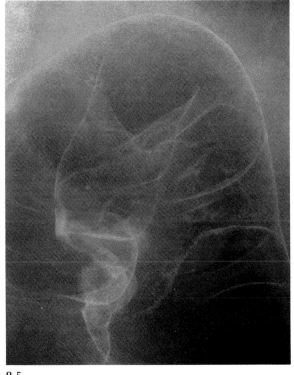

8.5

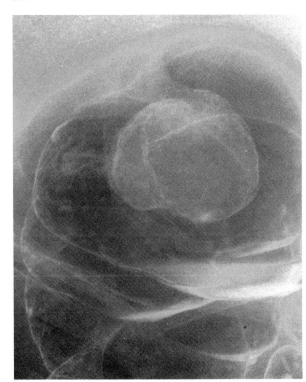

8.6

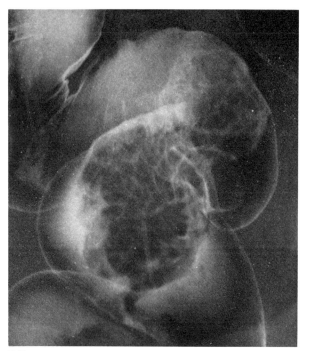

8.7a

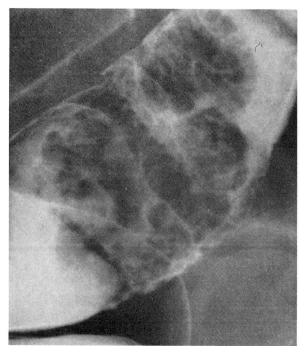

8.7b

8.7 **Villous adenomas** a,b
A large, irregular filling defect with a villous-type pattern is seen in the distal sigmoid colon. The patient, a 35-year-old female, complained of diarrhoea with a lot of mucus over a three-year period. Two sigmoidoscopic examinations and a barium enema performed two years previously at another hospital were negative. A sigmoid colectomy was performed; three villous adenomas were found on pathological examination but there was no evidence of malignancy

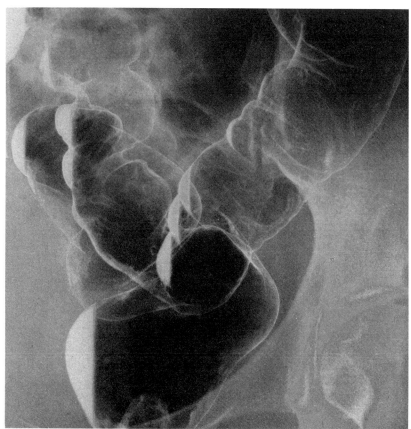

8.8

8.8 **Inflammatory polyps** Multiple small filiform polyps are seen in the sigmoid colon of a patient with a long history of ulcerative colitis

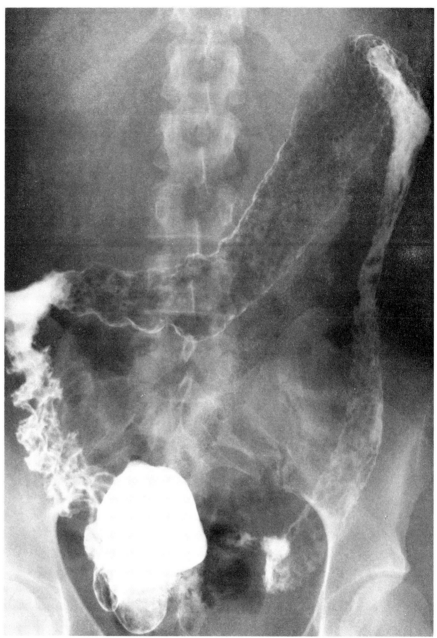

8.9

8.9 **Inflammatory polyps** A large number of polyps are seen throughout most of the colon in a patient with ulcerative colitis. Loss of the haustral pattern and shortening of the colon is also seen. The lumen of the descending and the sigmoid colon is narrowed

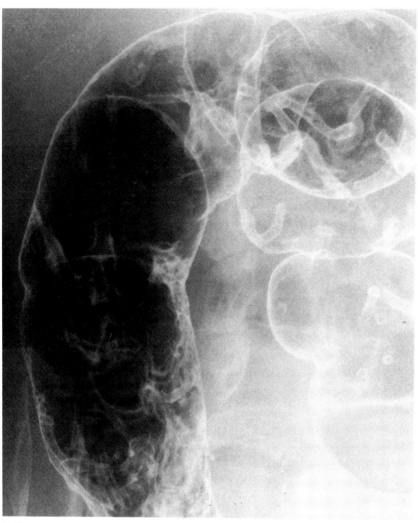

8.10

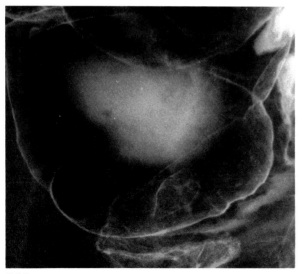

8.11

8.10 **Inflammatory polyps** Multiple large filiform polyps are seen in the hepatic flexure of a patient with a long history of ulcerative colitis

8.11 **Lipoma of the caecum** A small, slightly irregular, polypoid filling defect is shown in the caecal pole. It was removed at colonoscopy and proved to be a lipoma

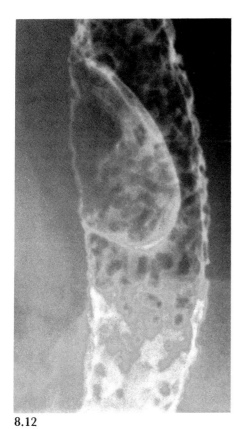

8.12

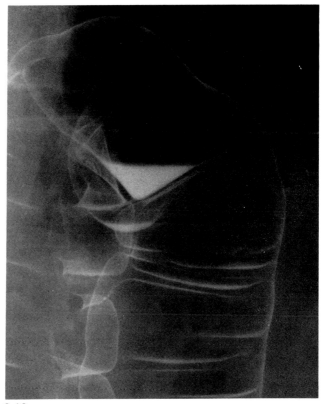

8.13

8.12 **Lipoma and ulcerative colitis** A smooth, rounded filling defect is seen occupying most of the lumen of a segment of the descending colon. There is loss of the haustral pattern and a moderate degree of mucosal ulceration. The patient was known to have had ulcerative colitis for some years and the barium examination was performed because of recurrence of symptoms. The polypoid lesion was removed at colonoscopy and proved to be a lipoma

8.13 **Hyperplastic polyp** A small oval filling defect is seen on a haustral fold in the descending limb of the splenic flexure. The polyp was removed at colonoscopy and proved to be a hyperplastic polyp on histological examination

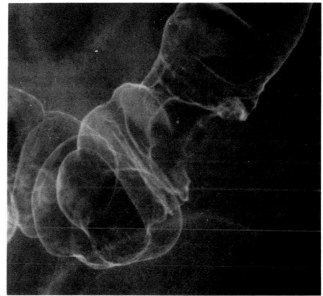

8.14

8.14 **Infiltrating carcinoma** Asymmetrical infiltration of a segment of sigmoid colon by tumour is seen. The patient presented with a six-month history of rectal bleeding. Examination of the resected specimen proved it was an invasive carcinoma

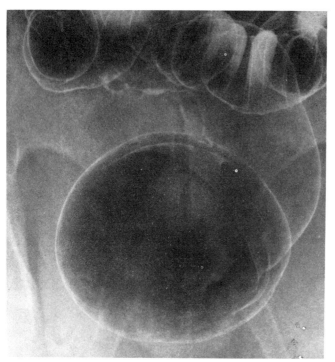

8.15

8.15 **Infiltrating carcinoma** This 50-year-old man presented complaining of blood on the surface of the motions. Five years previously he had a number of adenomatous polyps removed from the rectum. A sigmoidoscopic examination was performed before the barium enema but no lesion was seen. An irregular, infiltrating lesion of the right side of the distal sigmoid colon was shown on only this one *angled view*. At operation a carcinoma was found that proved to be a well-differentiated adenocarcinoma—Dukes 'B'

8.16 **Infiltrating carcinoma** An irregular, infiltrating lesion with narrowing of the lumen, destruction of the mucosa and shouldering of the margins is seen in the sigmoid colon. The patient who presented with constipation stated that his motions had become narrower and smaller. At operation an adenocarcinoma—Dukes 'C'—was found

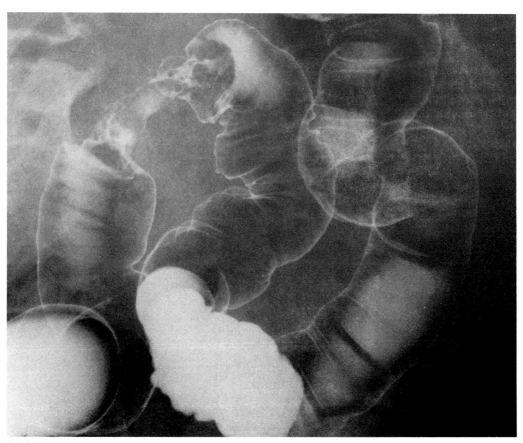

8.16

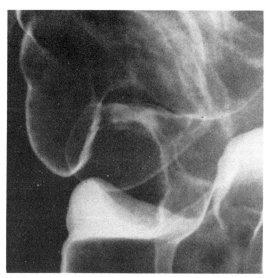

8.17

8.17 **Infiltrating carcinoma** A short 'apple-core' type deformity of the ascending colon is seen. The patient, a 68-year-old female, presented with iron deficiency anaemia. An adenocarcinoma—Dukes 'C'—was found at operation

8.18 **Carcinoma of the caecum** A slightly irregular infiltrating lesion is seen involving the medial aspect of the inverted caecum. The patient, a 44-year-old female, presented with right upper quadrant pain. Carcinoma was suggested on the barium enema report as being most likely to cause the caecal filling defect. Two colonoscopy examinations were carried out but no evidence of caecal carcinoma was found. The patient returned nine months later and a barium meal examination showed an infiltrating lesion of the second part of the duodenum (Figure 6.39). A carcinoma of the caecum invading the duodenum was found at operation. In retrospect it seems likely that the inverted caecum was not visualized at the colonoscopy examinations

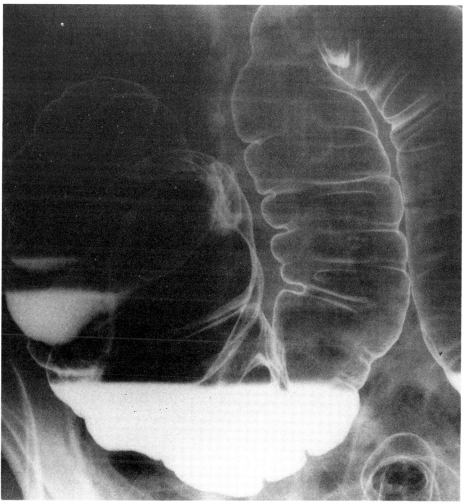

8.18

8.19 **Infiltrating carcinoma** A
single-contrast barium enema shows an
infiltrating carcinoma of the
ascending colon. The lesion was
suspected on double-contrast
examination but there was poor
mucosal coating. A single-contrast
examination was performed to
confirm the diagnosis and it showed
the lesion clearly. Better detail of the
caecum and ascending colon can
sometimes be obtained with dilute
barium than with a poorly coated
double-contrast examination

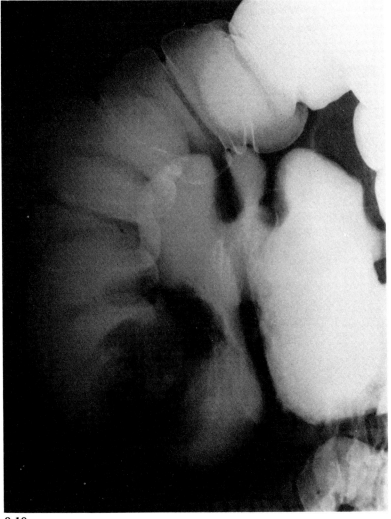

8.19

8.20 **Polypoid carcinoma of the sigmoid
colon** A barium enema performed three weeks
before this examination showed a filling defect in the
sigmoid colon, thought to be possibly faecal residue.
This *spot view* taken at the repeat examination shows
a slightly irregular polypoid filling defect, about
3 cm in diameter, confirming that the filling defect is
constant. Subsequent examination of the resected
specimen showed a well-differentiated
adenocarcinoma infiltrating into the inner margin of
the muscle layer but no deeper. Polypoid
carcinomas are sometimes overlooked because they
are considered to represent residual faecal material.
In this case the remainder of the colon was clean on
both occasions; a solitary lump of faecal residue is
an unlikely finding

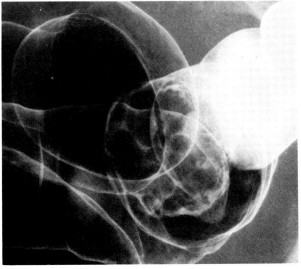

8.20

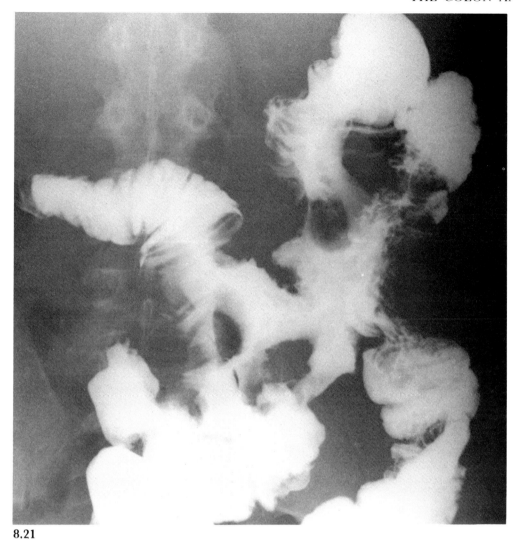

8.21

8.21 Carcinoma with coloenteric fistulae A
barium enema demonstrates an extensive carcinoma of
the transverse colon infiltrating adjacent loops of
small intestine in a 53-year-old man who presented
with abdominal pain, weight loss and anaemia

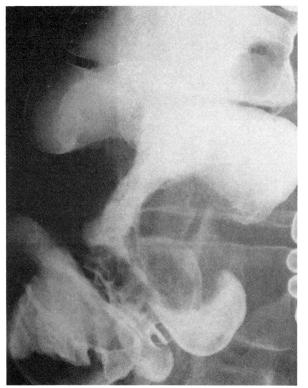

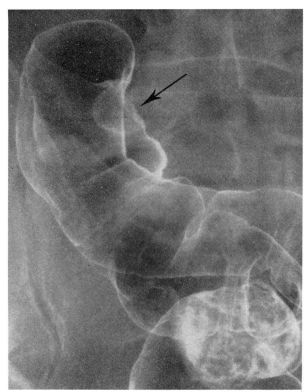

8.22a   8.22b

8.22 **Carcinoma and adenomatous polyps** a A large infiltrating adenocarcinoma of the caecum with marked narrowing of the lumen and shouldering of the margins is seen. b Two polyps, one pedunculated and the other sessile (arrow), are also seen in the sigmoid colon and proved to be tubulovillous adenomas

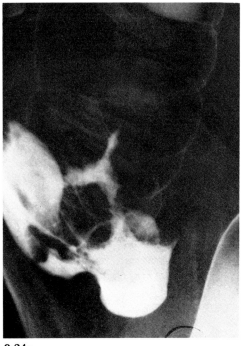

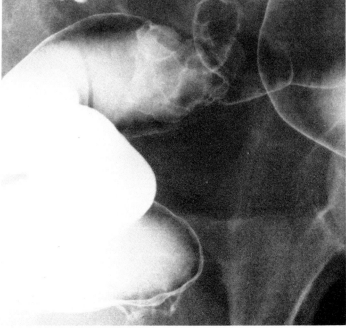

8.24a   8.24b

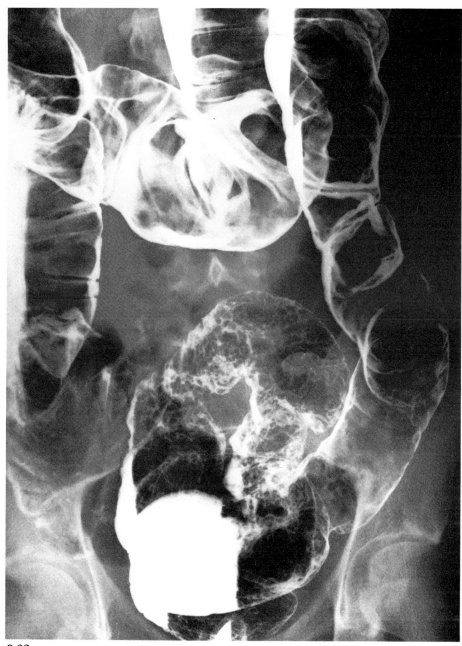

8.23

8.23 **Familial polyposis coli and carcinoma** Multiple polypoid filling defects are seen carpeting the sigmoid colon and rectum and there is a narrowed segment in the distal sigmoid colon. A large number of sessile polyps can also be seen in the transverse and descending colon. The patient, a 28-year-old man, presented with a two-year history of diarrhoea and a three-month history of abdominal pain. At sigmoidoscopy multiple polyps and a carcinoma were seen. Multiple metastases were found in the liver at operation. A left hemicolectomy was performed and three carcinomas, as well as a large number of polyps were found

8.24 **Two synchronous carcinomas** The patient presented with abdominal pain, weight loss and rectal bleeding. a There is gross distortion of the caecum by a large mass. b A further large irregular polypoid lesion is seen in the distal sigmoid colon. The presence of two carcinomas was confirmed at operation and there were hepatic metastases

8.25 **Carcinoma and ulcerative colitis** The patient, a 78-year-old female with a history of ulcerative colitis, was examined because of recurrence of symptoms. Changes were shown representing chronic ulcerative colitis involving most of the colon. This *spot view* of the sigmoid colon also shows a polypoid defect which proved to be a well-differentiated adenocarcinoma—Dukes 'A'

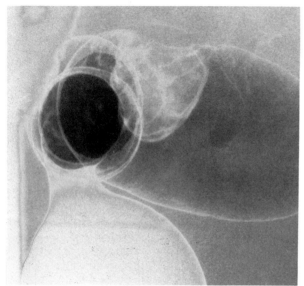

8.25

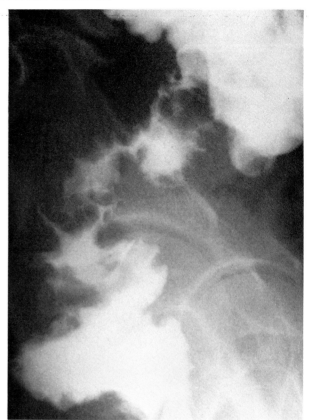

8.27

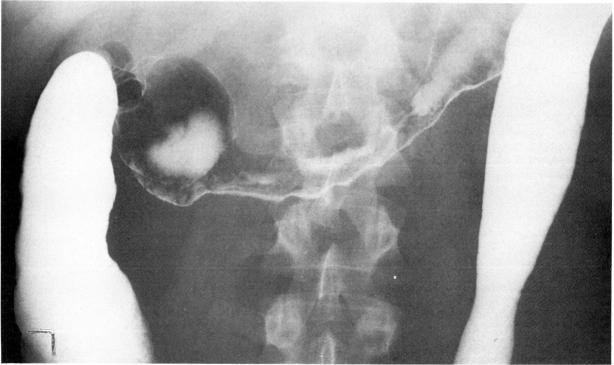

8.26

8.27 **Lymphosarcoma** A long irregular infiltrating lesion is seen distorting and narrowing the lumen of the distal sigmoid colon and the proximal part of the rectum. The patient presented with a two-month history of abdominal pain and diarrhoea. Fleshy material was seen on sigmoidoscopy; a biopsy taken showed evidence of lymphosarcoma on histological examination. Six months previously the patient had been investigated for hepatosplenomegaly but no cause was found

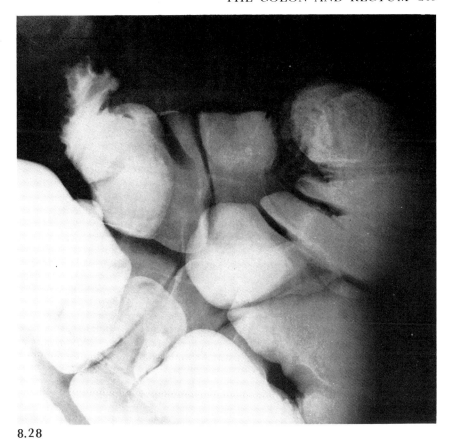

8.28

8.26 **Carcinoma and ulcerative colitis** An extensive infiltrating carcinoma is seen in the transverse colon. Changes of chronic ulcerative colitis were present throughout the remainder of the colon. The patient, a 40-year-old man, presented with weight loss and recurrence of bloody diarrhoea. A carcinoma extending from the hepatic flexure to the splenic flexure was confirmed at operation. It was adherent to the pancreas, inoperable, and many seedlings were present in the peritoneum. Histology of the peritoneal seedlings showed a poorly differentiated mucus-secreting adenocarcinoma

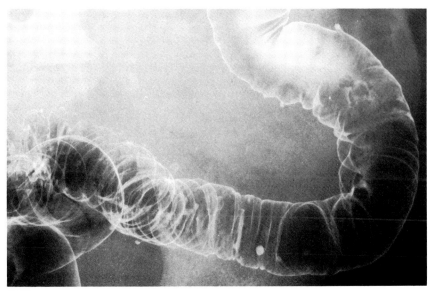

8.29

8.28 **Metastatic disease involving the transverse colon** A narrowed segment of the transverse colon is shown causing obstruction to the flow of barium. The patient, an 83-year-old female, was known to have carcinoma of the stomach

8.29 **Sigmoid diverticula** Multiple small diverticula are seen *en face* and in profile in the sigmoid colon. There is evidence of hypertrophy of the circular muscle

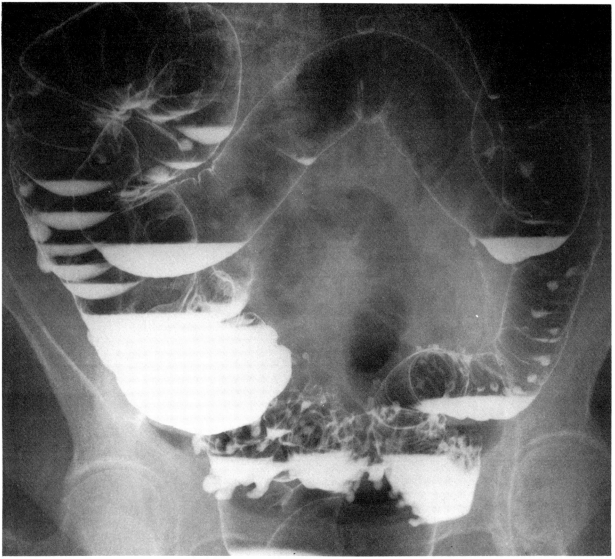

8.30

8.30 **Multiple colonic diverticula** Diverticula are seen
scattered throughout the colon; a large number are present in
the sigmoid colon

8.31 **A diverticulum** This *spot view* shows barium in a
diverticulum. The outer border of the barium outlining the
diverticulum is rounded and sharply defined

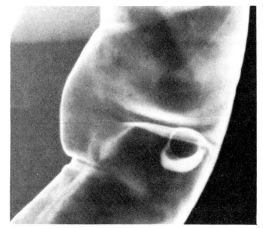

8.31

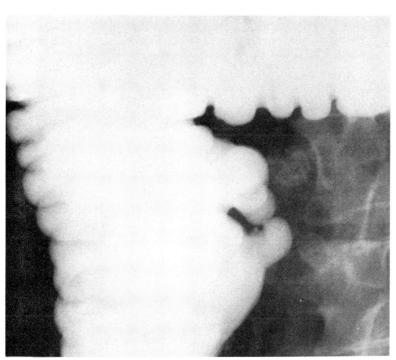

8.32

8.32 **Traction diverticula** Two diverticula, one quite large, are seen in the ascending colon adherent to calcified mesenteric lymph glands

8.33 **Diverticular abscess** A small irregular mass is seen indenting the lower margin of the sigmoid colon in a patient with diverticular disease. Two narrow tracks of barium, presumably the site of perforated diverticula, are seen passing into the mass

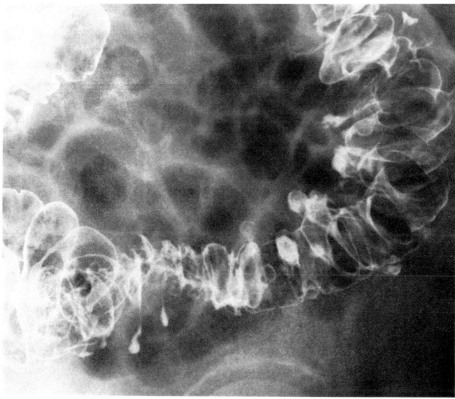

8.33

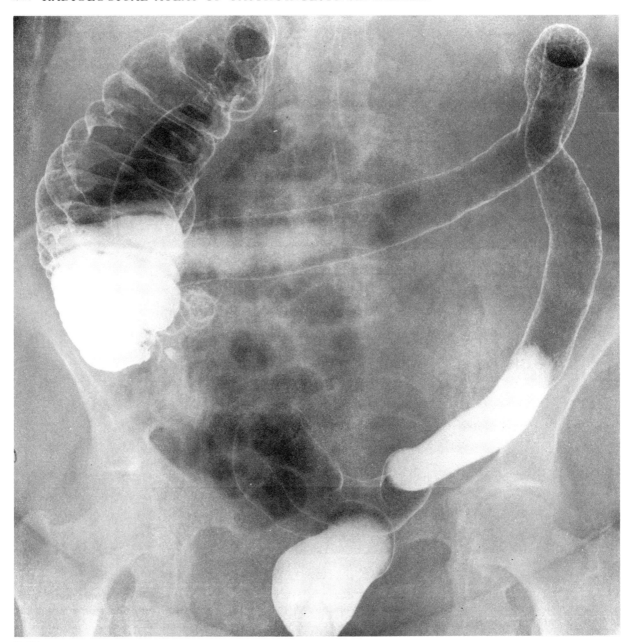

8.43

8.43 **Chronic ulcerative colitis** There is loss of the haustral pattern and shortening and narrowing of the transverse, descending and sigmoid colon as well as the rectum. The granular pattern of the mucosa indicates that the disease is active

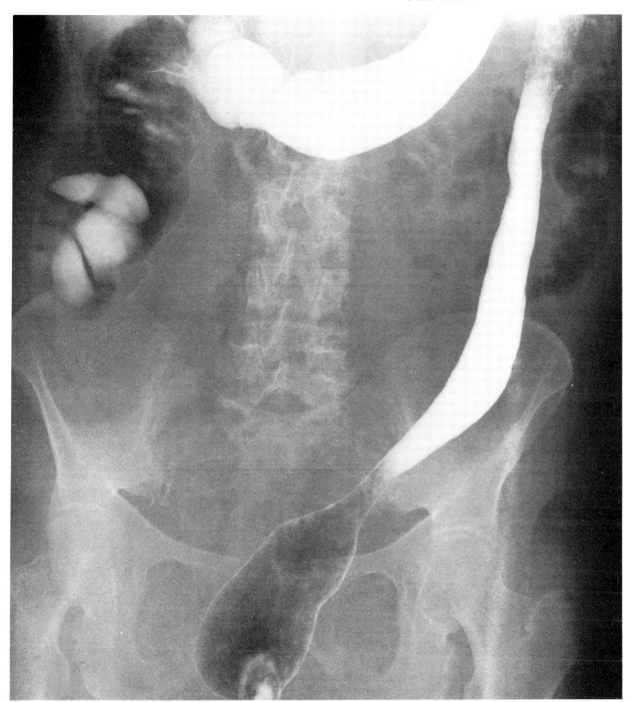

8.44a

8.44 **Chronic ulcerative colitis** a Considerable shortening of the sigmoid colon and descending colon is noted. There is narrowing of the lumen, particularly in the sigmoid colon.

8.44b The *lateral view* shows an increase in the presacral space. Oedema is often given as the reason for increase in the presacral space but it is more likely that it results from shortening of the sigmoid colon and rectum

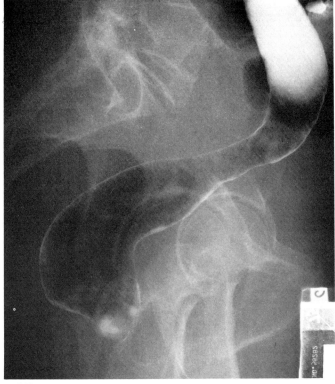

8.45 **Ulcerative colitis** Moderate mucosal ulceration is shown. There is also loss of the haustral pattern and shortening

8.44b

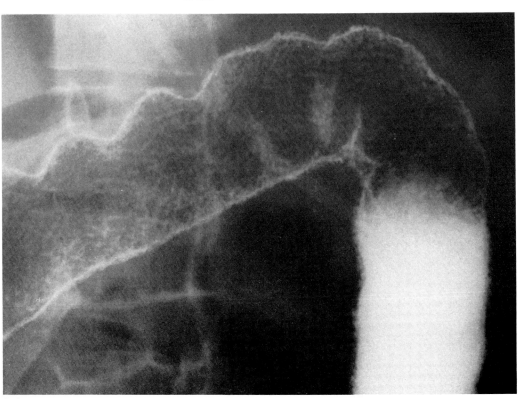

8.45

8.46 **Ulcerative colitis** A *double-contrast enema* shows the granular pattern of mild active ulcerative colitis

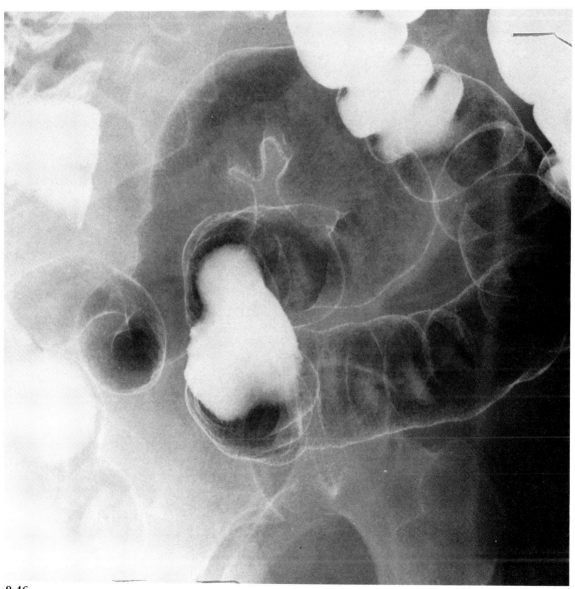

8.46

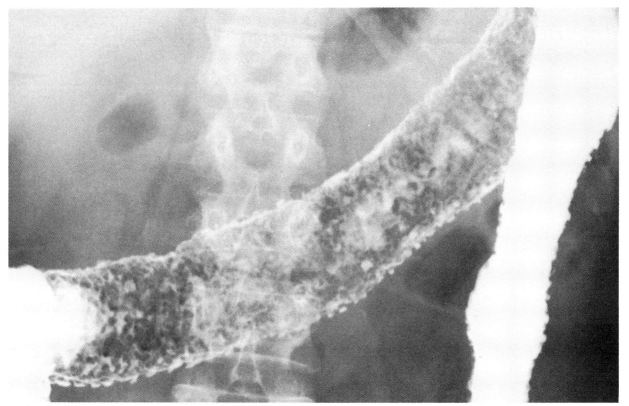

8.47

8.47 **Ulcerative colitis** Moderately severe mucosal ulceration and loss of the normal haustral pattern are shown

8.48 **Stricture in ulcerative colitis** A short tight stricture is seen at the rectosigmoid junction in a patient with a long history of ulcerative colitis

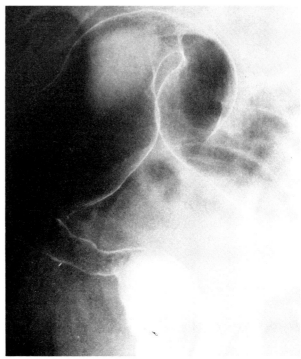

8.48

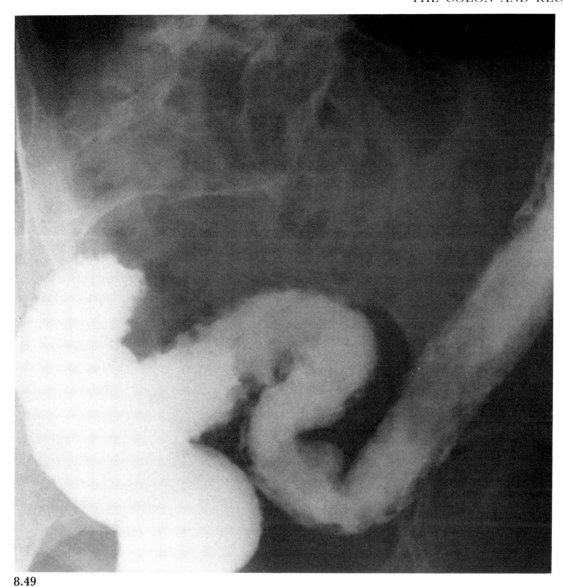

8.49

8.49 **Ulcerative colitis** Severe mucosal ulceration shown on a *single-contrast barium enema*. Multiple 'collar-stud' ulcers are present; in some places they join up and give a double contour to the outline of the colon

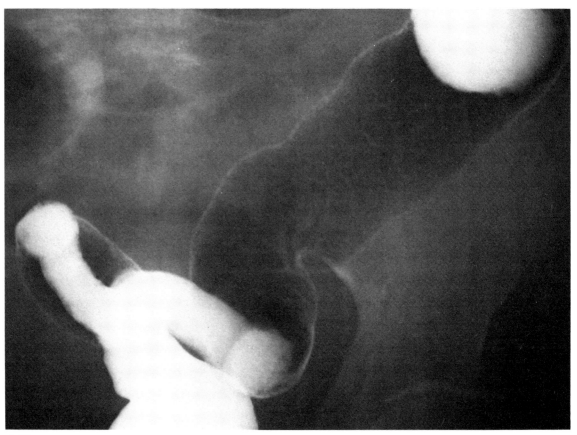

8.50

8.50 **Epithelial dysplasia in ulcerative colitis** There is an irregular nodular area in the sigmoid colon and colonic dysplasia in the mid sigmoid colon of an 84-year-old woman with a long history of ulcerative colitis. Two carcinomas of the ascending colon were also shown at this examination. Patients with severe dysplasia have a high risk of developing cancer

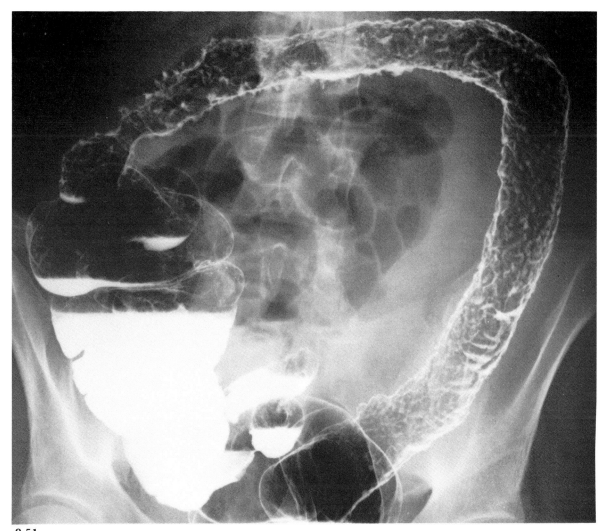

8.51

8.51 **Crohn's disease** Loss of the haustral pattern, shortening, and some narrowing and ulceration of the hepatic flexure, transverse colon, descending colon and proximal sigmoid colon are shown. A number of deep fissure ulcers are seen, particularly at the hepatic flexure. Transverse stripes are seen at the junction of the descending colon and the sigmoid colon. There is evidence of thickening of the wall of the descending and proximal sigmoid colon as shown by displacement of the gas-filled loops of small intestine. The distal sigmoid colon and rectum are not involved and there is relative sparing of the ascending colon. A barium study of the small intestine was also performed which showed evidence of Crohn's disease of the distal ileum

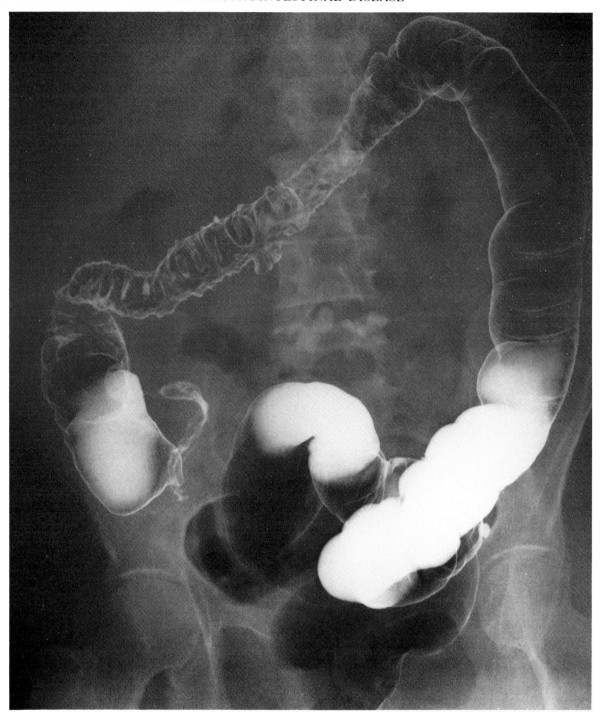

8.52a

8.52 **Crohn's disease** a Most of the right half of
the colon is abnormal and shows shortening,
narrowing, ulceration, transverse stripes and
asymmetry. There is no evidence of inflammatory
bowel disease in the descending colon, sigmoid colon
or rectum. b The terminal ileum is narrowed and
there is indentation of the medial wall of the caecum
by the thickened wall of the terminal ileum.
Otherwise the caecum and the proximal part of the
ascending colon are normal

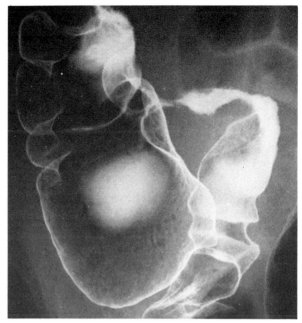

8.52b

8.53 **Discrete ulcers in Crohn's
disease** Multiple small collections of barium with a
surrounding zone of translucency are shown. The
mucosal pattern between the ulcers is normal

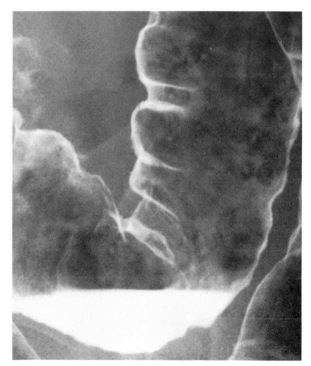

8.53

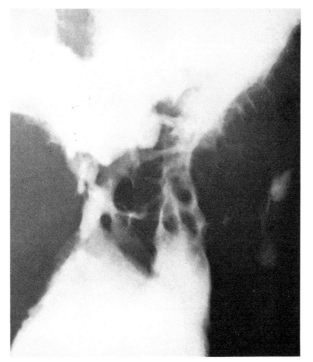

8.58

8.58 Fissure ulcers and sinuses in Crohn's disease There is gross distortion and narrowing of a.segment of descending colon with multiple sinuses leading to small abscess cavities. A number of deep fissure ulcers can also be seen

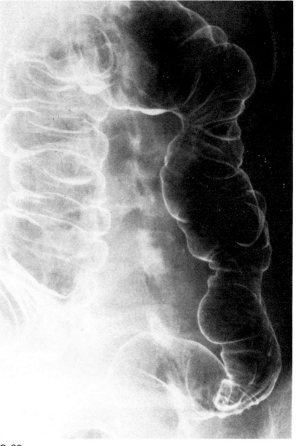

8.60

8.60 Asymmetry in Crohn's disease Small areas of involvement with Crohn's disease have resulted in contraction and pseudodiverticula formation

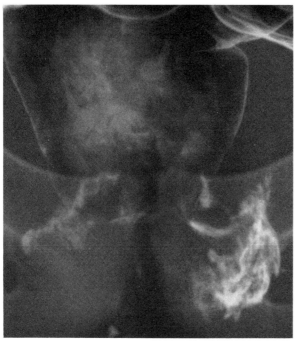

8.59

8.59 Perianal sinuses in Crohn's disease Multiple perianal sinuses are outlined with barium and there is an abscess cavity shown on the left side. The patient, a 22-year-old man, presented with severe perianal pain. At rectal examination a fleshy polypoid lesion was palpated on the posterior wall of the rectum and anal canal. A mass was detected in the right iliac fossa on palpation. Sigmoidoscopic examination was normal. Barium studies also confirmed the presence of ileocaecal Crohn's disease. The perianal and ischiorectal abscesses were drained at operation

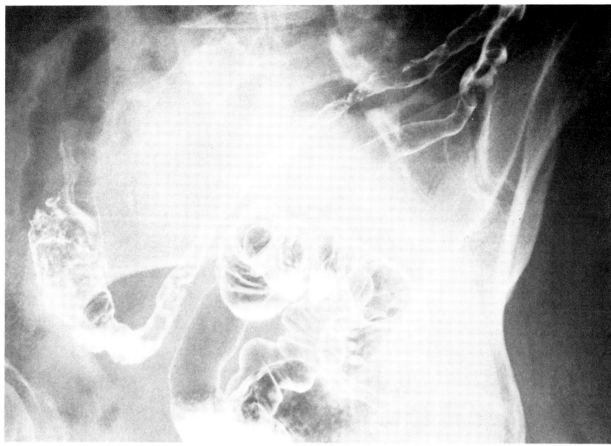

8.61

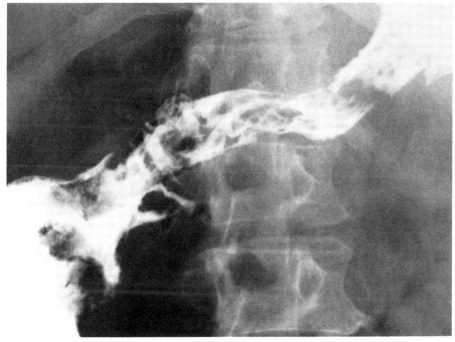

8.62

8.61 Stricture in Crohn's disease A long tight stricture of the transverse and descending colon is seen in a patient with a split ileostomy for Crohn's disease of the terminal ileum and colon

8.62 Carcinoma complicating Crohn's disease Multiple sinus tracks are shown at the proximal end of a narrowed segment of transverse colon. A number of inflammatory polyps are seen. At operation an extensive carcinoma was found which had not been suspected

8.66 Lymphogranuloma venerium
There is marked narrowing and shortening of the sigmoid colon and rectum. The 46-year-old Jamaican woman presented with a 4-month history of constipation and tenesmus. A tight rectal stricture was found on rectal examination. Lymphogranuloma venerium compliment fixation texts were positive. (Courtesy of Dr. Tom Walker)

8.67 Pseudomembranous enterocolitis A view of the sigmoid colon shows a markedly irregular outline to the colonic margin and multiple nodular defects in the barium column. Similar appearances were present throughout the remainder of the colon. The patient, an 85-year-old female, developed diarrhoea with blood and mucus following a course of ampicillin for a wound infection after sigmoid colectomy

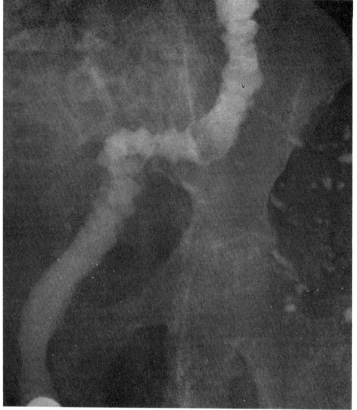

8.66

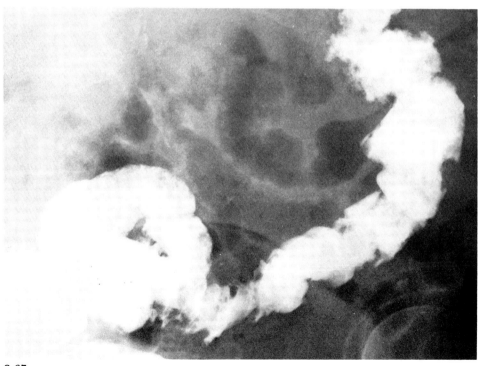

8.67

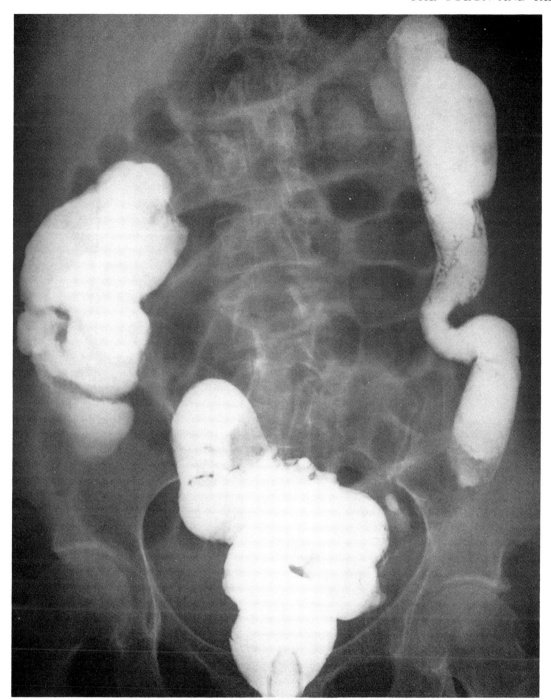

8.68

8.68 **Pseudomembranous enterocolitis** A serrated margin is present throughout the colon and there are multiple irregular defects in the barium, probably due to the presence of pseudomembrane. The patient, a 67-year-old female, developed diarrhoea with mucus following a course of cloxacillin prescribed to cover the skin grafting of a varicose ulcer (Nolan *et al.* 1976)

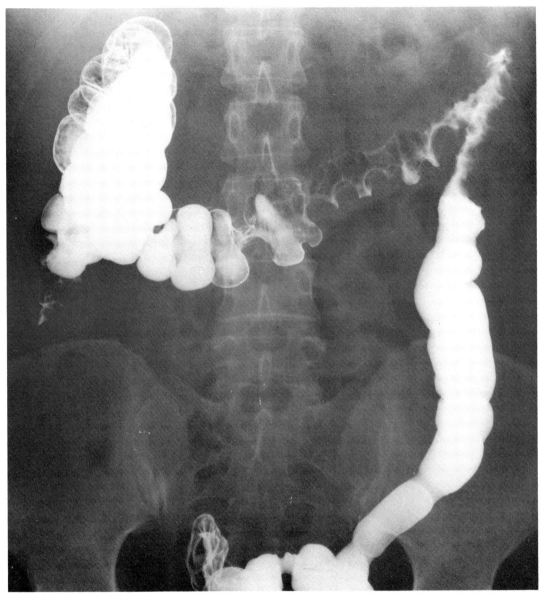

8.69

8.69 **Ischaemic colitis** The changes are limited to the splenic flexure where there is narrowing, some shortening and mucosal oedema giving the characteristic 'thumb-printing' appearance. The 43-year-old female patient presented with acute abdominal pain and rectal bleeding. The abnormal segments had returned to normal at a repeat examination two months later

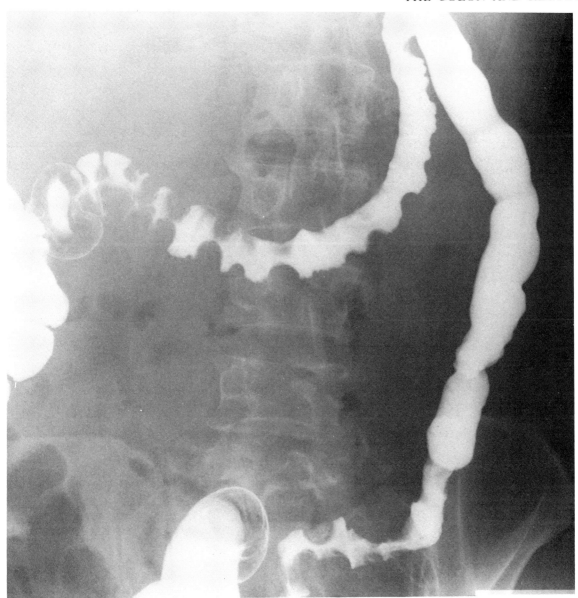

8.70

8.70 **Ischaemic colitis** The patient, a 54-year-old female, gave a ten-day history of loose motions and rectal bleeding with some pain. The clinical history was not typical of ischaemic colitis. The diagnosis was suggested on the barium enema which shows oedema with 'thumb-printing' in the transverse colon and the proximal sigmoid colon. Most of the descending colon has a featureless outline. It seems likely that the ischaemic process started at the splenic flexure and progressed to involve most of the colon. A further barium enema performed six weeks later showed that the colon had returned to normal

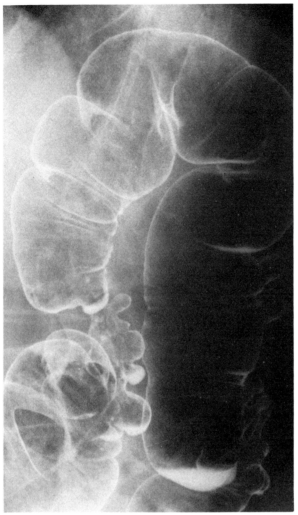

8.71

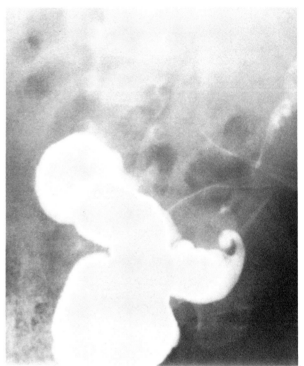

8.72

8.71 **Ischaemic stricture** A short asymmetrical segment of narrowing is seen in the ascending limb of the splenic flexure. A number of diverticula can also be seen in the descending colon. The 76-year-old woman presented with abdominal pain. Following this examination the narrowed segment was resected and proved to be an ischaemic stricture

8.72 **Necrotizing enterocolitis stricture** A long tight stricture of the distal descending and proximal sigmoid colon is seen in a two-month-old baby with a history of neonatal necrotizing enterocolitis

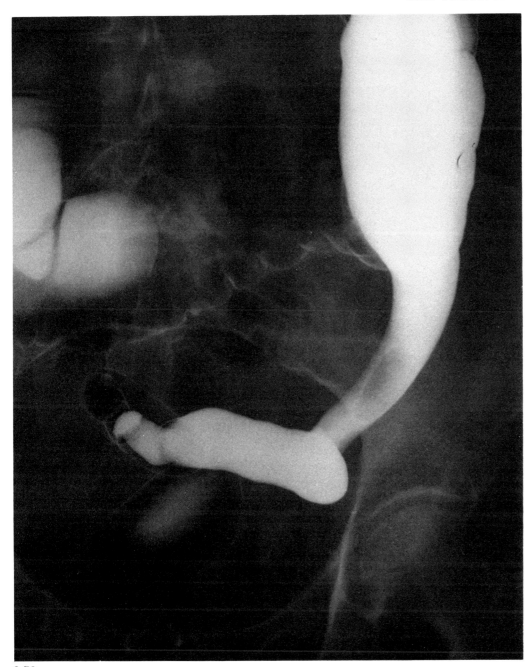

8.73

8.73 **Radiation colitis** The sigmoid colon is narrowed and shortened in a patient with a history of a hysterectomy and radiotherapy for carcinoma of the uterus. Histological examination of a rectal biopsy showed the typical changes of radiation damage

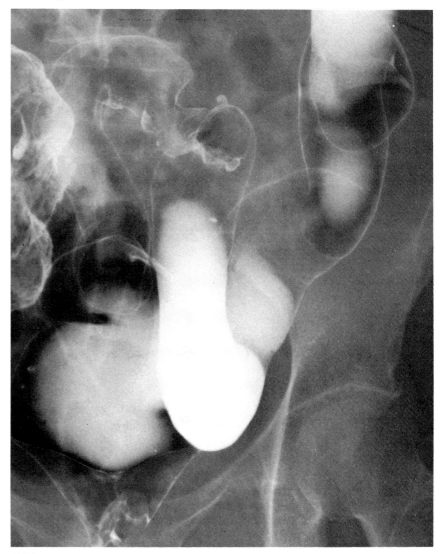

8.74

8.74 **Endometriosis** Smooth indentation and narrowing of a segment of sigmoid colon is seen with some adjacent diverticula in a 55-year-old woman with long-established endometriosis

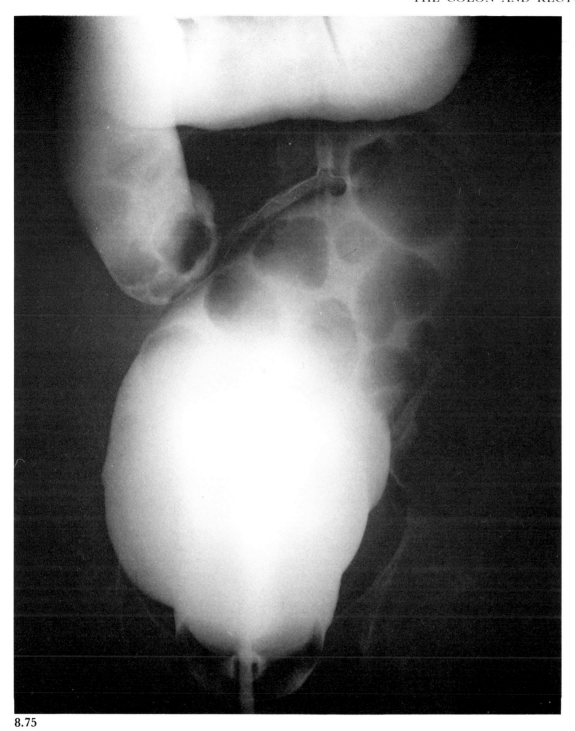

8.75

8.75 **Idiopathic megacolon** There is gross dilatation of the distal sigmoid colon and rectum

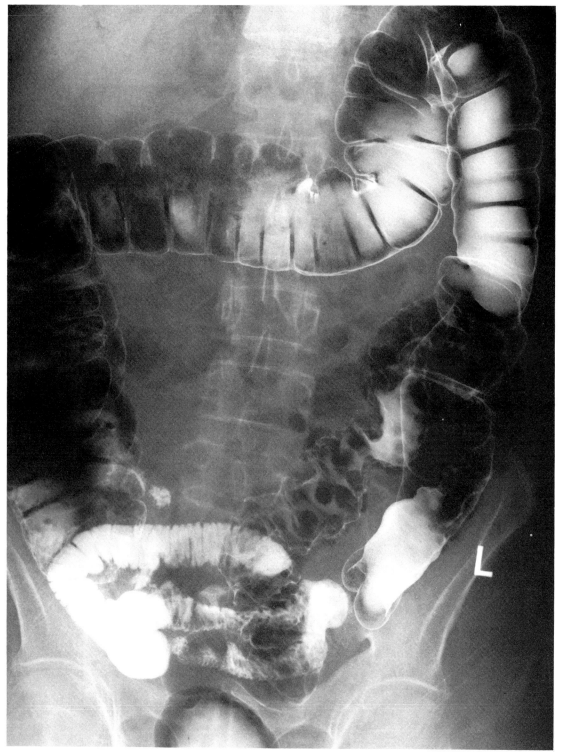

8.76

8.76 **Pneumatosis coli** a A large number of round gas-filled cysts can be seen in the wall of the sigmoid colon. b A detailed view of a short segment of sigmoid colon. This man presented with a history of diarrhoea and passing mucus

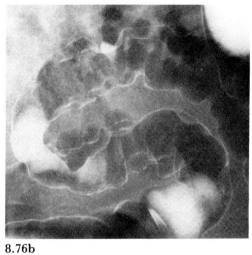

8.76b

8.77 **Cathartic colon** There is loss of the normal haustral pattern of the colon with almost complete absence of the hepatic and splenic flexures. Dilatation of the terminal ileum and proximal half of the colon is also seen. (Courtesy of Dr. J.T.J. Privett)

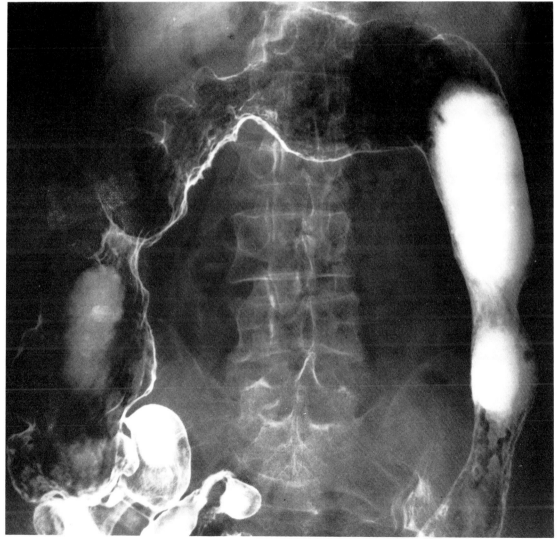

8.77

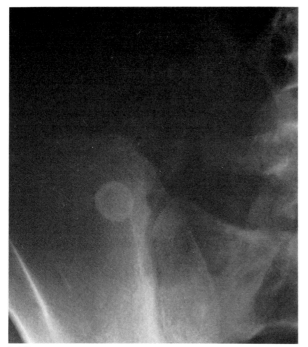

8.78a

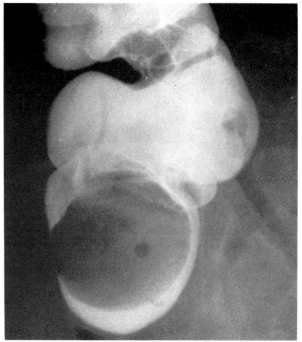

8.79

8.79 **Mucocele of the appendix** A round well-defined filling defect is seen in the caecum with non-filling of the appendix. The small round translucent area in the centre of the larger mass represents the proximal end of the appendix which is not dilated and has not filled with barium. This was an incidental finding on a barium study performed for investigation of ulcerative colitis. At operation a mucocele of the appendix was confirmed (Nolan 1977)

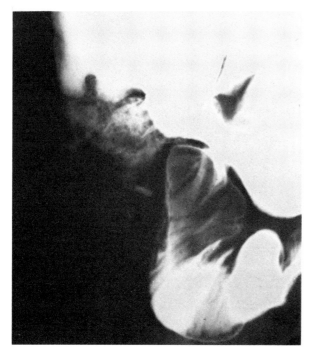

8.78b

8.78 **Appendix calculus and appendicitis** a A round calculus is seen in the right lower quadrant of a young man who was admitted with lower abdominal pain. b A *barium enema* shows the calculus obstructing the lumen of the appendix. An appendix calculus with associated acute appendicitis was found at operation

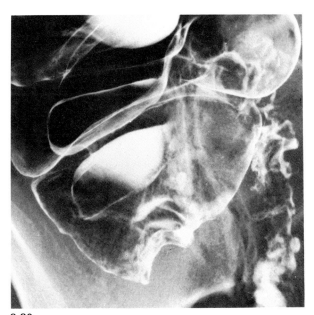

8.80

8.80 **Appendix stump** A small indentation is shown at the caecal pole. This was constant and showed no change at a repeat examination 16 months later. The patient had had a previous appendicectomy

Despite advances in other imaging techniques it is surprising how often gastrointestinal angiography still produces the definitive answer in a difficult diagnostic problem. It is likely that both the quality and safety of angiography will increase with the development of digital vascular imaging systems and non-ionic contrast media, and these factors, together with an increasing therapeutic role, seem likely to ensure that visceral angiography will continue to play an important part in the management of gastrointestinal disorders.

Angiography of the gastrointestinal tract is performed for either the diagnosis or therapy of gastrointestinal bleeding, the evaluation or management of portal hypertension and occasionally, the pre-operative localization, pre-operative assessment, or therapy of gastrointestinal tumours (Baum *et al.* 1965; Reuter & Bookstein 1968; Athanasoulis *et al.* 1976; Allison 1980a). Good gastrointestinal angiography requires a fairly experienced radiologist, adequate equipment with the facility for exposing radiographs both in rapid sequence and for a sufficient period following a contrast injection, a mechanical injection pump for the rapid delivery of contrast medium, and high-quality radiography. Although it is perfectly feasible to perform visceral angiography on an occasional basis, the interpretation of the radiographs is at least as difficult as the angiographic technique, and there is little doubt that the reliability and diagnostic value of the procedure is greatest in those units where it is performed regularly.

The three major vessels of supply to the alimentary tract are the coeliac axis, the superior mesenteric artery and the inferior mesenteric artery. Although all three vessels fill with an abdominal aortic injection, the radiographic detail on such a study is inadequate for diagnosis and it is usually desirable to perform selective studies of the major vessels and/or superselective studies of branch vessels. The selection of visceral vessels to be studied, and their sequence of investigation will obviously be influenced by the clinical situation: in a case of haematemesis, for instance, interest would be focussed on the coeliac and superior mesenteric territories rather than the inferior mesenteric. Details of angiographic techniques in the gastrointestinal tract are to be found in the literature (Abrams 1971), and will not be considered further here.

The coeliac axis

Adequate opacification of the coeliac territory is normally achieved in the adult patient with 30–50 ml of contrast medium (Urografin 370* or equivalent) delivered at 8–10 ml/sec by a mechanical injector. For superselective studies a hand injection is sufficient. The radiographic filming sequence should extend sufficiently long to allow visualization of the portal venous system in the late films. In most patients this occurs between 8 and 14 seconds after the injection; it may take longer, however, and filming should continue up to 20 seconds if this is possible. In the capillary phase of the coeliac study the dense

---

* Sodium diatrizoate 0.1 g/ml + meglumine diatrizoate 0.66 g/ml, Schering Chemicals Limited, FRG

9 Angiography of the Gastrointestinal Tract

D.J. Allison and A.P. Hemingway

opacification of normal structures may be mistaken for a pathological lesion such as a tumour. This error is particularly likely to occur in respect of the mucosa of the fundus of the stomach and the duodenal cap and can be obviated by preliminary distension of these organs with carbon dioxide gas.

The tail of the normal pancreas may also appear dense because of foreshortening in the AP projection; doubts about this area may be resolved by a study in the right posterior oblique projection. The value of angiography in the coeliac territory in identifying pathology is very dependent on the nature of the lesion. Vascular tumours or malformations are usually easy to identify but other lesions such as peptic ulcers which cause minimal morphological changes in the vasculature are usually impossible to demonstrate unless they are actively bleeding during the angiographic procedure, or have produced secondary changes in vessels such as aneurysms.

Diagnostic angiography to localize a source of acute bleeding is performed if endoscopy has failed to identify a bleeding site; extravasation of as little as 0.5 ml/min can be shown on selective angiography (Frey et al. 1970), and in the authors' experience the technique is successful in 90 per cent of patients with clinical evidence of ongoing bleeding.

Angiography is sometimes undertaken with the specific object of embolizing bleeding vessels in patients who are unsuitable for emergency surgery (Rosch et al. 1972). Single vessels such as the left gastric, gastroduodenal or gastroepiploic arteries can be embolized with relative impunity owing to the rich collateral circulation available in the upper gastrointestinal tract (Allison 1978). Gastric (Goldman et al. 1976) and duodenal (Shapiro et al. 1981) necrosis have both been reported, however, following therapeutic embolization of coeliac branches and particular care should be exercised when artheroma is present, or there has been previous surgery which may have compromised potential sources of collateral circulation. Therapeutic embolization is especially useful in the emergency management of bleeding into the biliary tree; such cases are very difficult to manage surgically owing to the problem of localizing the source of bleeding, and the morbidity associated with hepatic surgery. Sometimes the embolization obviates the need for surgery altogether; for example, in some cases of bleeding secondary to trauma, hepatic biopsy, or previous biliary surgery.

Considerable variations occur in the normal vascular anatomy of the coeliac axis. These most frequently affect the origins of the hepatic arteries, and the

commonest variations are described in the legend to Figure 9.6. The venous drainage of the coeliac territory is of particular importance in the assessment of portal hypertension; visualization of the portal venous system may establish the site of obstruction, demonstrate the routes of collateral drainage (e.g. varices), and gives information relating to portal haemodynamics which may affect management decisions concerning shunt surgery.

Therapeutic embolization may also be employed in the portal venous circulation, either to obliterate varices (Lunderquist & Vang 1974; Dick 1981), or to occlude the transhepatic catheter track as a prophylactic manoeuvre following transhepatic portal venous sampling for the localization of hormone-producing tumours of the pancreas.

The superior mesenteric artery

The superior mesenteric artery is usually easy to catheterize selectively and requires 30–50 ml of contrast medium (Urografin 370) delivered at 8–12 ml/sec for adequate opacification in the adult patient. Care should be taken to include the caecum and ascending colon in the radiographic field since these are likely sites for angiodysplasia to be found (Baum et al. 1977; Boley et al. 1977; Allison 1980a). It is also important to continue the filming sequence up to 20 seconds after the injection of contrast medium. This allows opacification of the portal system or the sites of abnormal venous collaterals if portal hypertension is present. It also ensures that abnormal venous filling from tumours or angiodysplasia is demonstrated and that extravasated contrast in the case of active bleeding can be visualized. In the case of small bowel lesions, which may be difficult to localize surgically, or which are found in patients who have previously undergone negative laparotomies, considerable assistance can be given to the surgeon by selectively catheterizing the branch artery supplying the lesion and performing intraoperative angiography.

A disease which is often responsible for occult gastrointestinal bleeding is angiodysplasia. This disorder consists of abnormalities in the microcirculation of the mucous and submucous layers of the bowel wall, usually in the caecum and ascending colon (Baum et al. 1977; Boley et al. 1977). Angiography is particularly important in the diagnosis of angiodysplasia because the tiny lesions comprising the disorder are often difficult to demonstrate by other diagnostic techniques. Although the diagnosis can be made by an experienced endoscopist, other methods including barium studies, isotope studies and even laparotomy, are usually incapable of identifying the lesions.

The inferior mesenteric artery

The inferior mesenteric artery is the most difficult of the three major visceral vessels to catheterize. The calibre of the vessel is smaller than the coeliac or superior mesenteric vessels. A hand injection is usually sufficient to achieve adequate opacification. Foreshortening of the sigmoid colon produces overlapping vascular shadows in the AP projection, and detail of this section of bowel is best obtained by a study in the left posterior oblique projection. For the same reason detailed views of the splenic flexure are best obtained on an oblique view; in this case, however, the best projection is a right posterior oblique study because of the colonic anatomy in this region. In clinical practice the diagnostic return from inferior mesenteric angiography is less than that obtained from coeliac or superior mesenteric studies.

References

Abrams H.L. (1971) *Angiography*. Boston: Little, Brown & Company

Allison D.J. (1978) Therapeutic embolization. *Br. J. Hosp. Med.*, **20**, 707

Allison D.J. (1980a) Gastrointestinal bleeding: radiological diagnosis. *Br. J. Hosp. Med.*, **23**, 359

Allison D.J. (1980b). Therapeutic embolization and venous sampling. In *Recent Advances in Surgery* (Ed. Taylor S.). London: Churchill Livingstone

Allison D.J. (1983) Interventional radiology. In *Recent Advances in Radiology and Diagnostic Imaging* (Ed. Steiner R.E.). London: Churchill Livingstone

Athanasoulis C.A., Waltman A.C., Novelline R.A., Krudy A.G. & Sniderman K.W. (1976) Angiography: its contribution to the emergency management of gastrointestinal haemorrhage. *Radiol. Clin. North Am.*, **14**, 265

Baum S., Nusbaum M., Blakemore W.S. & Finkelstein A.K. (1965) The pre-operative radiographic demonstration of intra-abdominal bleeding from undetermined sites by percutaneous selective coeliac and superior mesenteric arteriography. *Surgery*, **58**, 797

Baum S., Athanasoulis C.A., Waltman A.C., Galdabini J., Schapiro R.H., Warshaw A.L. & Ottinger L.W. (1977) Angiodysplasia of the right colon; a cause of gastrointestinal bleeding. *Am. J. Roentgenol.*, **129**, 789

Boley S.J., Sammartano R., Adams A., DiBiase A., Kleinhaus S. & Sprayregen S. (1977) On the nature and aetiology of vascular ectasias of the colon (degenerative lesions of ageing). *Gastroenterology*, **72**, 650

Dick R. (1981) Transhepatic injection of varices. *Br. J. Hosp. Med.*, **26**, 340

Forbes W. St. C., Nolan D.J., Fletcher E.W.L. & Lee E. (1978) Small bowel melaena: 2 cases diagnosed by angiography. *Br. J. Surg.*, **65**, 168

Frey C.F., Reuter S.R. & Bookstein J.J. (1970) Localization of gastrointestinal haemorrhage by selective angiography. *Surgery*, **67**, 548

Goldman N.L., Land W.C., Bradley E.L. & Anderson J. (1976) Transhepatic therapeutic embolization in the management of massive upper gastrointestinal bleeding. *Radiology*, **120**, 340

Lunderquist A. & Vang J. (1974) Transhepatic catheterization and obliteration of the coronary vein in patients with portal hypertension and oesophageal varices. *N. Engl. J. Med.*, **291**, 646

Nebesar R.A., Kornblith P.L., Pollard J.L. & Michels N.A. (1969) *Coeliac and Superior Mesenteric Arteries*. London: J. & A. Churchill

Reuter S.R. & Bookstein J.J. (1968) Angiographic localization of gastrointestinal bleeding. Gastroenterology, **54**, 876

Rosch J., Dotter C.T. & Brown M.J. (1972) Selective arterial embolization. A new method for control of acute gastrointestinal bleeding. *Radiology*, **102**, 303

Shapiro N., Brandt L., Sprayregan S., Mitsudo S. & Giotzer P. (1981) Duodenal infarction after therapeutic gelfoam embolization of a bleeding duodenal ulcer. *Gastroenterology*, **80**, 176

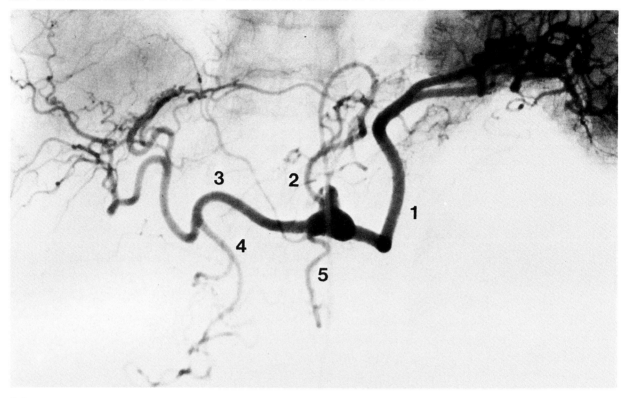

9.1

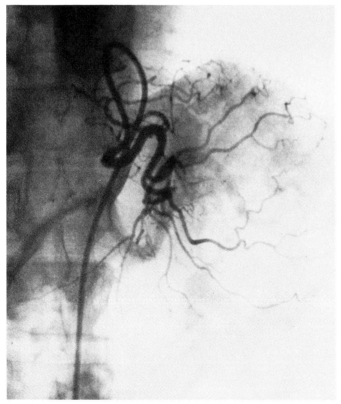

9.2

9.1 *Coeliac angiogram—normal anatomy*
1 splenic artery, *2* left gastric artery,
3 hepatic artery, *4* gastroduodenal artery,
5 dorsal pancreatic artery

9.2 *Selective left gastric angiogram—normal anatomy* Note the branch vessels coursing over the fundus and body towards the greater curvature

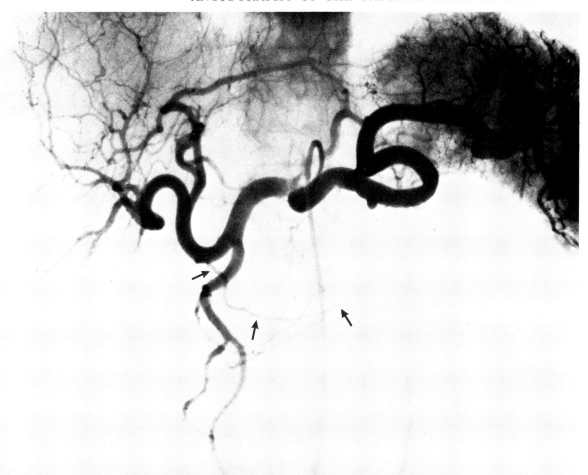

9.3

9.3 *Coeliac angiogram—normal anatomy* The right gastric artery (arrows) is shown arising from the hepatic artery and coursing around the lesser curve of the stomach to link with the left gastric artery. The right gastric artery is not usually easy to identify at angiography

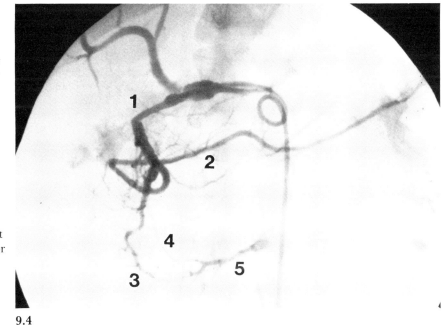

9.4 *Selective gastroduodenal angiogram—normal anatomy* 1 gastroduodenal trunk, 2 right gastroepiploic artery, 3 anterior superior pancreaticoduodenal artery, 4 posterior superior pancreaticoduodenal artery, 5 common inferior pancreaticoduodenal artery

9.4

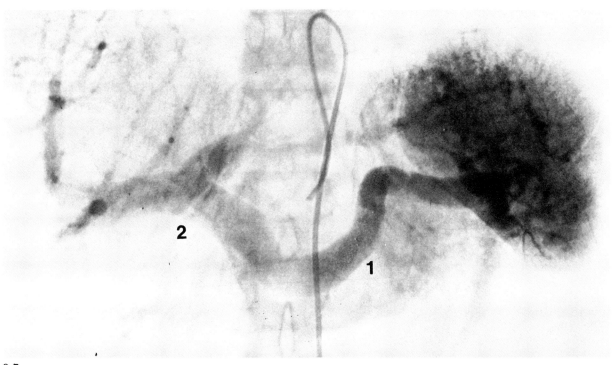

9.7

9.7 *Coeliac angiogram—venous phase* The indirect
splenoportogram shows normal portal venous
anatomy. *1* splenic vein, *2* portal vein dividing into
right and left main lobar branches.

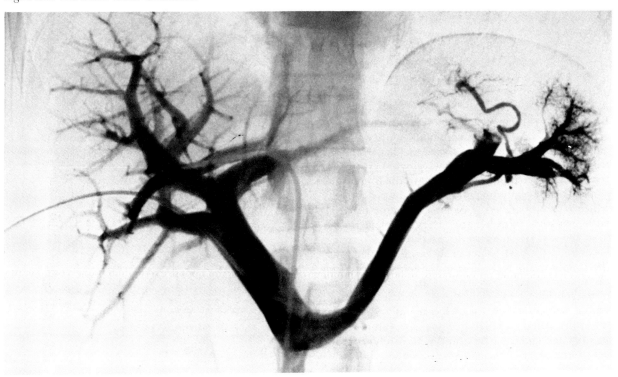

9.8

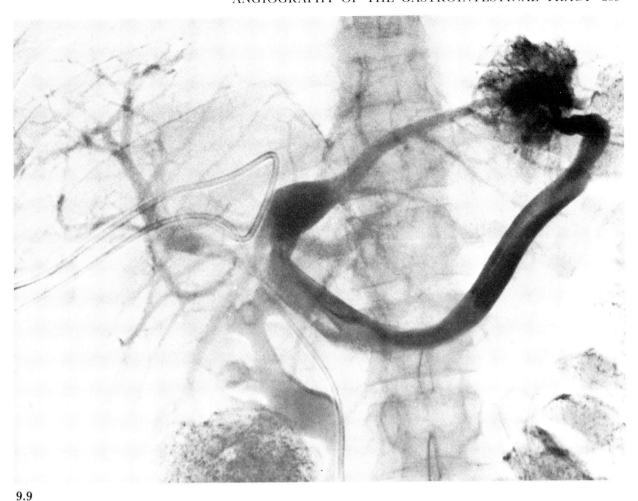

9.9

9.9 *Direct splenoportogram—trans-splenic approach* A
percutaneous puncture of the spleen gives direct
opacification of the portal venous system. This
procedure will probably become obsolete with the
advent of digital vascular imaging techniques

9.8 *Direct splenoportogram—transhepatic approach* A
percutaneous transhepatic puncture of the portal
vein gives catheter access for pancreatic venous
sampling or embolization of varices (Allison 1980b)

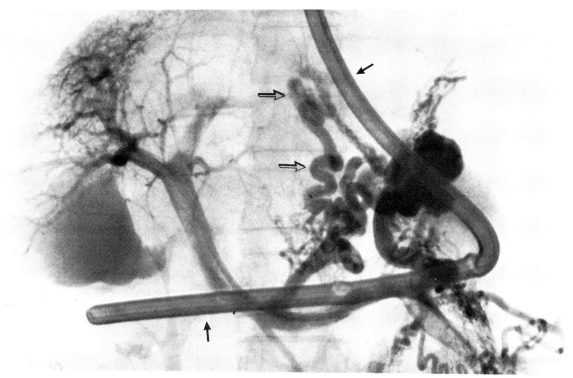

9.10a

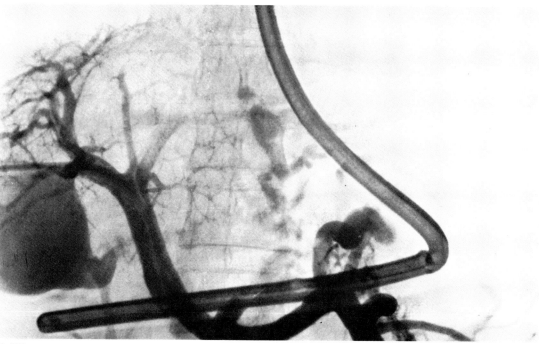

9.10b

9.10 **Gastric and oesophageal varices** a *Percutaneous transhepatic splenic portogram* The 56-year-old man had bleeding from oesophageal varices which was not controlled by a Sengstaken tube (single arrows). The portal vein was catheterized and the varices opacified (double arrows). Note the small cirrhotic liver. b *Embolization of varices* The varices have been embolized with isobutyl-2-cyanoacrylate

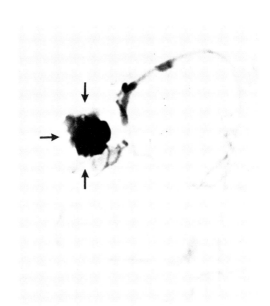

9.11a

9.11b

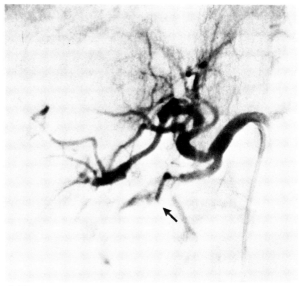

9.11c

9.11 **Embolization of duodenal ulcer** A 78-year-old woman with a bleeding diathesis presented with haematemesis, and a large bleeding duodenal ulcer was seen at endoscopy. It was decided to stop the bleeding using therapeutic embolization. a *Selective gastroduodenal angiogram* The contrast medium is outlining a large ulcer cavity (arrows). b A few seconds later the duodenal lumen has been opacified because of the brisk haemorrhage. c *Angiogram—post-embolization study* demonstrating the hepatic artery and the origin of the embolized gastroduodenal artery (arrow). The bleeding has stopped (Allison 1980a)

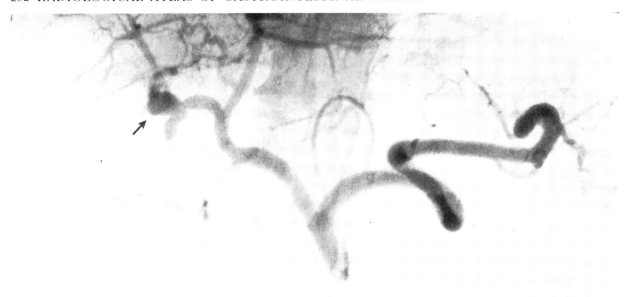

9.12a

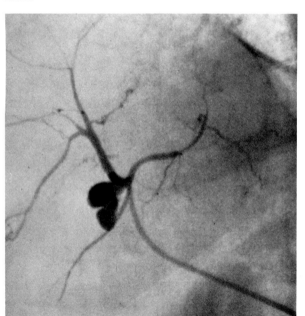

9.12b

9.12 **Embolization in a case of haemobilia** A man of 50 presented in shock with massive haemobilia following previous surgical damage to the hepatic artery and common bile duct. a *Coeliac angiogram* showing iatrogenic hepatic artery aneurysm (arrow). b *Superselective right hepatic angiogram* shows detail of aneurysm. c A few seconds after injection of the contrast it is seen leaking from the aneurysm into the common bile duct. d *Coeliac angiogram—post-embolization study* The hepatic artery is blocked with isobutyl-2-cyanoacrylate (arrow). The patient required no further treatment and was discharged from hospital one week later (Allison 1982)

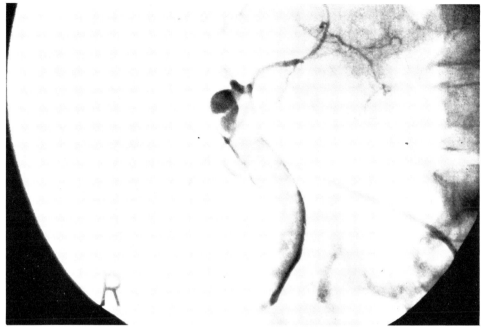

9.12c

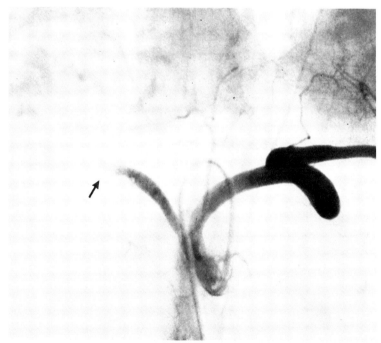

9.12d

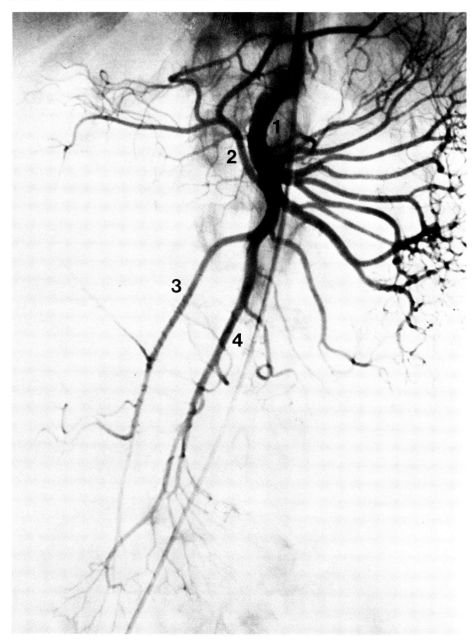

9.13a

9.13 *Superior mesenteric angiogram—normal anatomy* a *Arterial phase 1* main trunk,
2 common origin of right colic and middle colic arteries, *3* ileocolic artery,
4 continuation of superior mesenteric trunk giving rise to ileal branches and
eventually anastomosing with the ileocolic artery to form the ileocolic loop.
Branches to the jejunum arise from the main trunk of the superior mesenteric

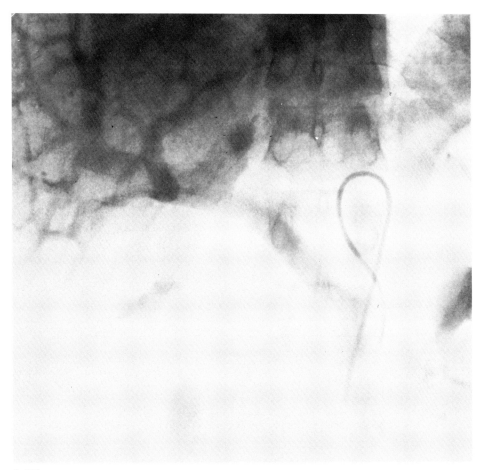

9.13b

artery proximal to the ileocolic origin. b *Venous phase* A late film in the
superior mesenteric study shows the portal venous system and is a good
alternative method to the indirect coeliac splenoportogram. Using two
catheters the coeliac and mesenteric venous systems can be opacified
simultaneously if desired

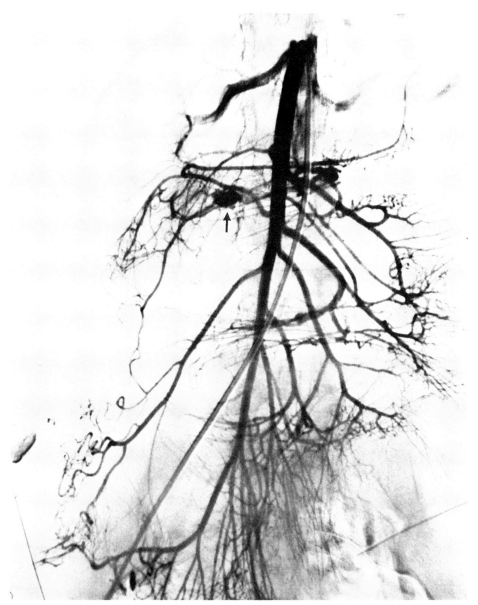

9.14a

9.14 **Jejunal arteriovenous malformation** A 26-year-old woman presented with a five-year history of anaemia and recurrent melaena. Numerous investigations including three laparotomies had failed to identify the bleeding site. a *Superior mesenteric angiogram* shows an abnormal vascular blush (arrow). b *Selective jejunal arteriogram—arterial phase* The first jejunal branch artery has been selectively injected and the lesion is opacified (arrow). c *Selective jejunal angiogram—venous phase* The vascular blush in the lesion and in the jejunal wall shows the abnormality to lie in the first loop of jejunum; this exact anatomical localization enabled the surgeon to resect the lesion, although the bowel appeared macroscopically normal. Histology showed the features of an arteriovenous malformation and the patient remains well two years later

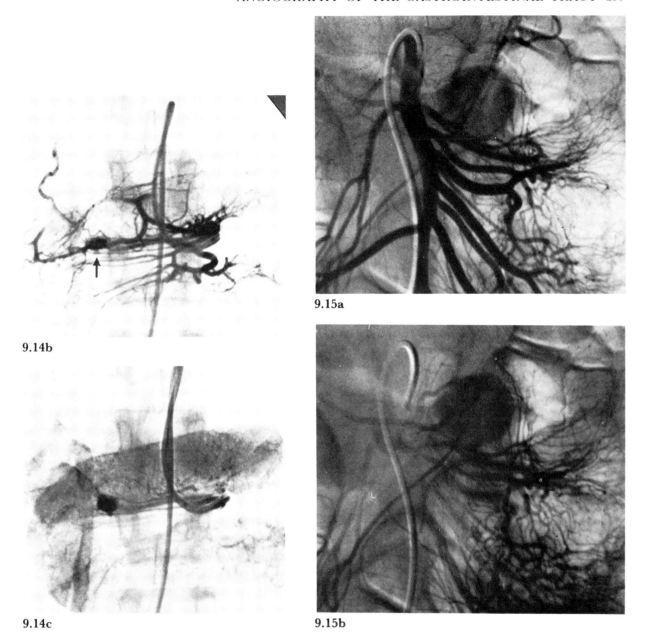

9.14b

9.14c

9.15a

9.15b

9.15 **Jejunal leiomyoma** a *Selective superior mesenteric angiogram* shows a round well-defined homogeneous vascular blush supplied mainly by the first jejunal branch. b Early draining veins can be seen in the *late arterial phase*. The 28-year-old woman presented one month before with melaena. Barium studies of the upper gastrointestinal tract showed no abnormality. She was discharged but 12 days later was readmitted with recurrence of melaena. Barium studies of the small intestine and colon were negative. At operation a mass, 3 cm × 2.5 cm, was found at the duodenojejunal flexure and resected. Histology proved it to be a leiomyoma (Forbes *et al.* 1978)

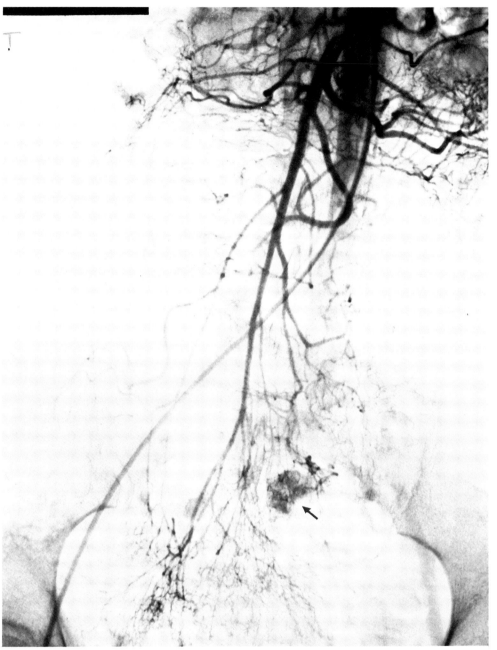

9.16a

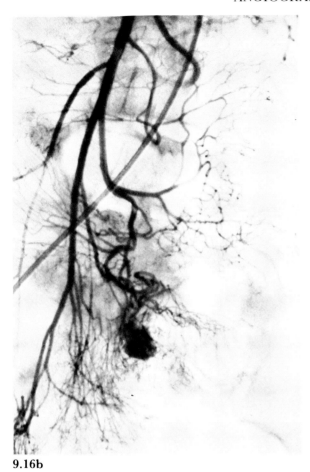

9.16b

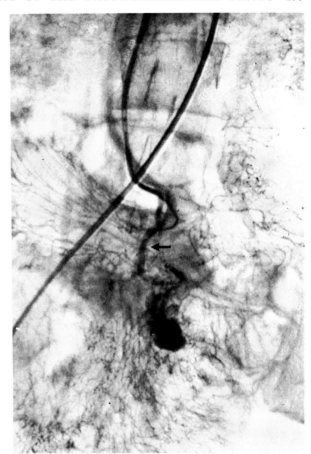

9.16c

9.16 **Ileal haemangioma** The 61-year-old woman presented with a two-year history of anaemia.
a *Superior mesenteric angiogram* There is an abnormal vascular blush in the upper ileum (arrow). b The catheter has been advanced into the vessel feeding the abnormal area, giving better detail of the lesion. c The *venous phase* of the superselective study shows a conspicuous vein draining the abnormal area (arrow). The angiographic appearances would suggest either a haemangioma or a vascular tumour such as a leiomyoma or a carcinoid tumour. To assist the surgeon the catheter was left in a superselective position and the patient transferred to the operating theatre. d An *intraoperative angiogram* confirmed the exact site of the tumour (arrow), permitting a limited resection of the abnormal bowel. Histology showed a polypoid cavernous haemangioma and the patient remains well two years later

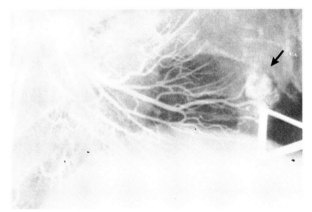

9.16d

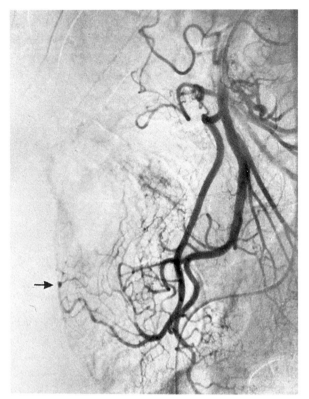

9.17a

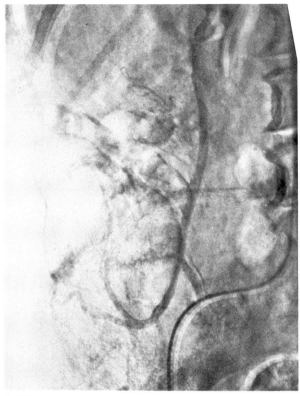

9.17b

9.17 **Colonic angiodysplasia** A 53-year-old man suffered from anaemia for 20 years. He had undergone two previous negative laparotomies.
a *Superior mesenteric angiogram* There is an abnormal vascular lake in the caecum (arrow). b The *capillary phase* of the study shows an early-filling conspicuous vein arising from the caecal lesion. c Injection of the resected specimen with a barium–gelatin mixture shows an area of angiodysplasia (arrow).
d *High-resolution microradiograph* (× 60) of normal bowel. e *High-resolution microradiograph* (× 60) of an area of angiodysplasia. Histological sections confirmed the angiographic diagnosis of angiodysplasia (Allison 1980a)

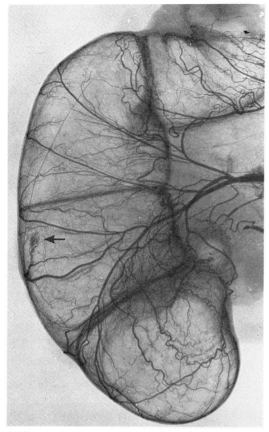

9.17c

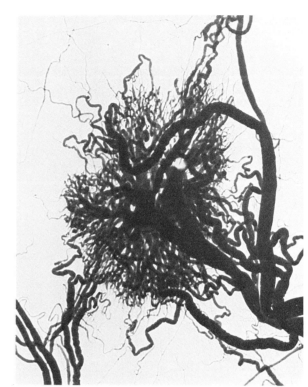

9.17e

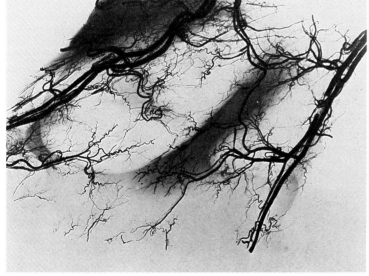

9.17d

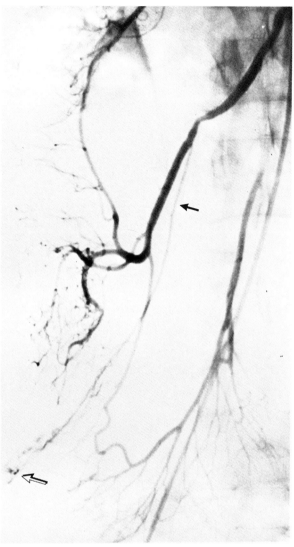

9.18a

9.18b

9.18 **Angiodysplasia of the appendix** A 19-year-old man presented with chronic gastrointestinal blood loss. a *Selective ileocolic angiogram* shows the appendicular artery (single arrow), and an abnormal vascular blush in the appendix (double arrow). b The *capillary phase* of the study shows areas of angiodysplasia in the caecum and appendix (arrows). Note the prominent appendicular vein (double arrow). The patient refused operation

9.19 **Mesenteric haemangioma** A woman of 58 presented with chronic anaemia and positive faecal occult blood tests. Endoscopy and barium studies revealed no gastrointestinal abnormality. a *Superior mesenteric angiogram—arterial phase* There is a large area of abnormal vascularity in the mesentery (arrows). b *Superior mesenteric angiogram—venous phase* There is a massive vein draining the abnormal area. At operation a vascular tumour was found in the mesentery. It had eroded into the jejunal wall causing intraluminal bleeding. Histology showed a benign haemangioma

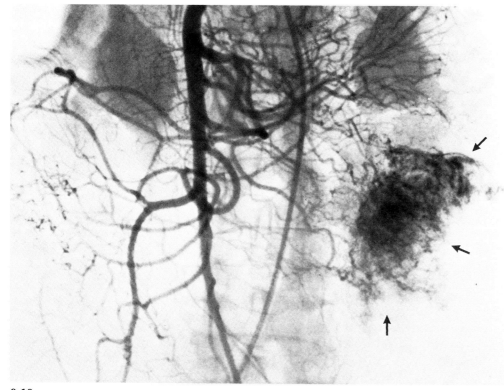

9.19a

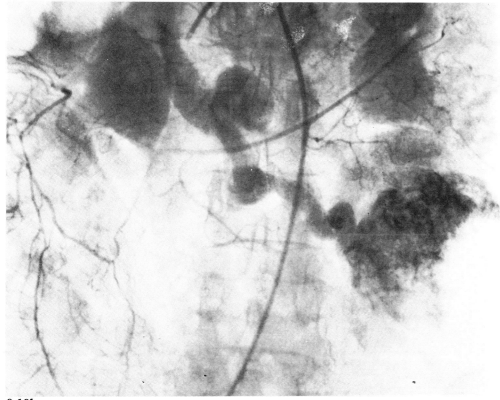

9.19b

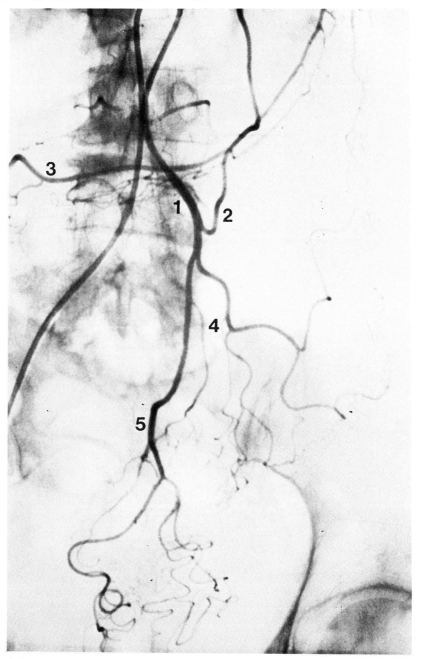

9.20a

9.20 *Inferior mesenteric angiogram—normal anatomy* a *AP projection 1* main trunk of the inferior mesenteric artery, *2* superior left colic artery, *3* middle colic artery (arising from superior mesenteric artery and anastomosing with superior left colic), *4* inferior left colic arteries,

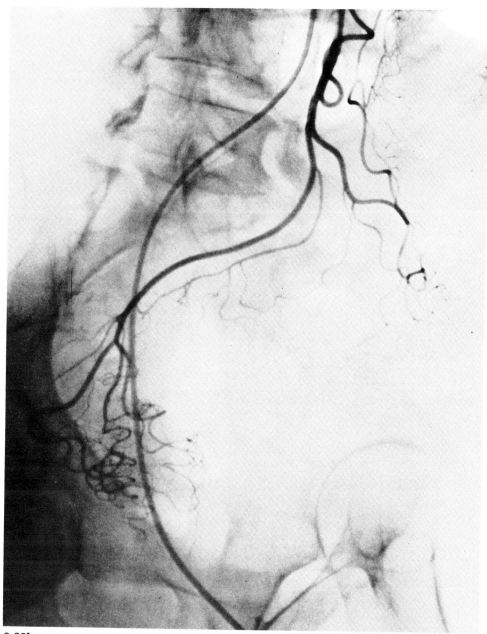

9.20b

5 superior rectal artery. b *Inferior mesenteric angiogram—normal anatomy*.
This *left posterior oblique projection* unfolds the sigmoid colon which is very
foreshortened in the AP projection

9.21 *Inferior mesenteric angiogram—normal anatomy* This study shows the anastomotic connection between the middle colic and superior left colic territories. Note how the retrograde filling of the middle colic artery has caused opacification of the superior mesenteric artery (arrow)

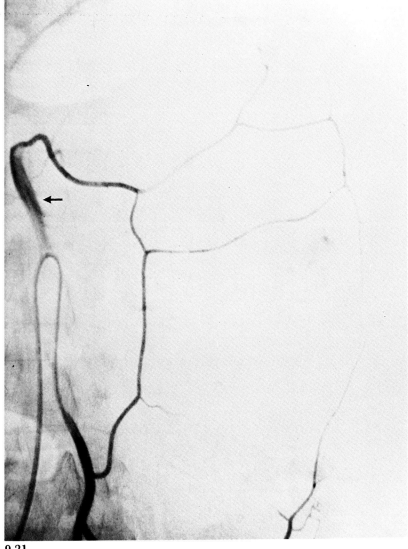

9.21

9.22 **Bleeding polyp in descending colon** A 60-year-old man presented with rectal bleeding. a The *arterial phase of an inferior mesenteric arteriogram* appears normal. b In the *venous phase* an abnormal vascular blush is seen in the descending colon, with extravasation of contrast medium into the lumen of the bowel (arrow). Note that the catheter has been deliberately flicked out of the inferior mesenteric artery between the arterial and venous phases of the study; this prevents wedging of the catheter in the small calibre vessel thereby ensuring that a good venous phase is obtained. At operation a benign polyp was resected from the descending colon (Allison 1980a)

9.23 **Carcinoma of the colon** A 55-year-old man presented with chronic anaemia. Angiodysplasia was suspected clinically. Previous barium enema and colonoscopy were said to be normal apart from diverticular disease. a *Arterial phase of the inferior mesenteric angiogram* appears normal. b The *venous phase* of the study shows an area of pathological circulation with a prominent draining vein (arrows). The appearances suggest a local inflammatory or neoplastic condition. The dense rounded shadow (double arrow) is barium in a diverticulum. Colonoscopy and biopsy showed the abnormal lesion to be a carcinomatous plaque

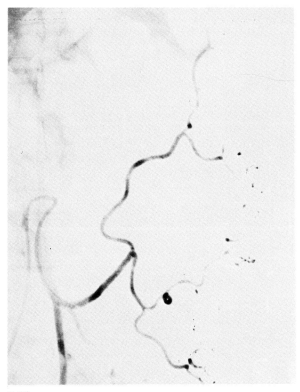

9.22a

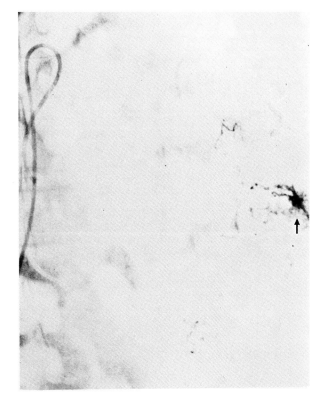

9.22b

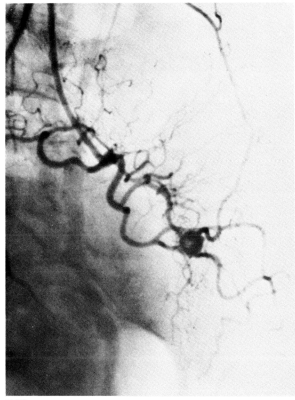

9.23a

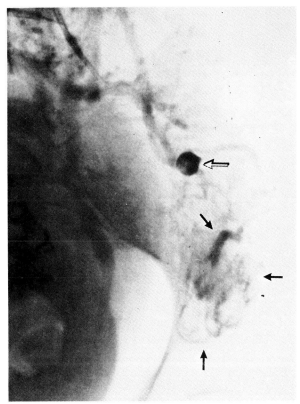

9.23b

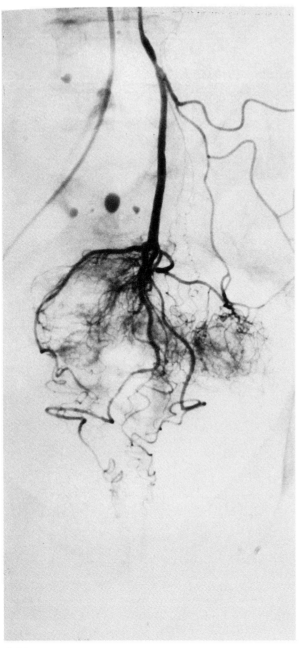

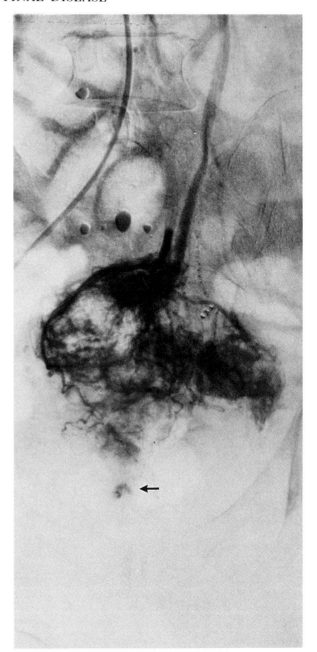

9.24a

9.24b

9.24 **Haemorrhoids** A 45-year-old woman was referred for angiography because of chronic anaemia. Physical examination and gastrointestinal investigations were said to reveal no abnormality. Coeliac and superior mesenteric angiograms were normal. a *Selective superior rectal angiogram—arterial phase* The appearances are within normal limits. b In the *capillary/venous phase* of the study the normal dense blush of the rectum is seen. In addition there is a blush in the anal canal—a characteristic angiographic finding in haemorrhoids (arrow). . Proctoscopy confirmed the diagnosis and the patient's haemorrhoids were treated. This is an invasive and expensive way of diagnosing piles which is not recommended by the authors!

Index